T0227241

Smile Design

Editors

BEHNAM BOHLULI
SHAHROKH C. BAGHERI
SEIED OMID KEYHAN

DENTAL CLINICS OF NORTH AMERICA

www.dental.theclinics.com

July 2022 • Volume 66 • Number 3

ELSEVIER

1600 John F. Kennedy Boulevard • Suite 1800 • Philadelphia, Pennsylvania, 19103-2899

http://www.dental.theclinics.com

DENTAL CLINICS OF NORTH AMERICA Volume 66, Number 3
July 2022 ISSN 0011-8532, ISBN: 978-0-323-98715-8

Editor: John Vassallo; j.vassallo@elsevier.com
Developmental Editor: Ann Gielou M. Posedio

Dental Clinics of North America (ISSN 0011-8532) is published quarterly by Elsevier Inc., 360 Park Avenue South, New York, NY 10010-1710. Months of issue are January, April, July, and October. Business and Editorial Offices: 1600 John F. Kennedy Boulevard, Suite 1800, Philadelphia, PA 19103-2899. Periodicals postage paid at New York, NY and additional mailing offices. Subscription prices are $323.00 per year (domestic individuals), $854.00 per year (domestic institutions), $100.00 per year (domestic students/residents), $377.00 per year (Canadian individuals), $863.00 per year (Canadian institutions), $100.00 per year (Canadian students/residents) $441.00 per year (international individuals), $863.00 per year (international institutions), and $200.00 per year (international students/residents). International air speed delivery is included in all *Clinics* subscription prices. All prices are subject to change without notice. **POSTMASTER:** Send address changes to *Dental Clinics of North America*, Elsevier Health Sciences Division, Subscription Customer Service, 3251 Riverport Lane, Maryland Heights, MO 63043. **Customer Service (orders, claims, online, change of address): Elsevier Health Sciences Division, Subscription Customer Service, 3251 Riverport Lane, Maryland Heights, MO 63043. Tel: 1-800-654-2452 (U.S. and Canada). Fax: 314-447-8029. E-mail: journalscustomerservice-usa@elsevier.com (for print support); journalsonlinesupport-usa@elsevier. com (for online support).**

Reprints. For copies of 100 or more, of articles in this publication, please contact the Commercial Reprints Department, Elsevier Inc., 360 Park Avenue South, New York, NY 10010-1710. Tel.: 212-633-3874; Fax: 212-633-3820; E-mail: reprints@elsevier.com.

The Dental Clinics of North America is covered in *MEDLINE/PubMed (Index Medicus), Current Contents/Clinical Medicine, ISI/BIOMED* and *Clinahl.*

Contributors

EDITORS

BEHNAM BOHLULI, DMD, OMFS, FRCD(C)
Clinical Instructor, Departement of Oral and Maxillofacial Surgery, University of Toronto, Toronto, Ontario, Canada

SHAHROKH C. BAGHERI, DMD, MD, FACS, FICD
Georgia Oral and Facial Reconstructive Surgery, Attending Oral and Maxillofacial Surgeon, Northside Hospital, Director of Fellowship Program in Facial Cosmetic and Reconstructive Surgery, Consultant, Council of Scientific Affairs, ADA

SEIED OMID KEYHAN, DDS, OMFS
Oral and Maxillofacial Surgeon, Founder and Director, Maxillofacial Surgery and Implantology, Biomaterial Research Foundation, Tehran, Iran; Co-Investigator, Department of Oral and Maxillofacial Surgery, College of Medicine, Jacksonville, Florida, USA

AUTHORS

KELVIN I. AFRASHTEHFAR, DDS, MSc, Dr, FDSRCS, FRCDC
Evidence-Based Practice Unit, Division of Restorative Dental Sciences, Clinical Sciences Department, College of Dentistry, Ajman University, Ajman City, UAE; Department of Reconstructive Dentistry & Gerodontology, School of Dental Medicine, Faculty of Medicine, University of Bern, Berne, Switzerland

ZAHRA AKBARI, MD
Private Practioner, Tehran, Iran

JORGE ALANIA, DDS
Private Practice, San Isidro, Lima, Peru

MARZIEH ALIKHASI, DDS, MS
Dental Research Center, Dentistry Research Institute, Tehran University of Medical Sciences, Tehran, Iran

BRIAN ALPERT, DDS, FACS, FACD, FICD†
Professor of Oral and Maxillofacial Surgery, University of Louisville, Louisville, Kentucky, USA

GHAZAL ANOOSH, DDS, MSc
Department of Periodontics, Faculty of Dentistry, Tehran Medical Sciences, Islamic Azad University, Tehran, Iran

BEHNAM BOHLULI, DMD, OMFS, FRCD(C)
Clinical Instructor, Oral and Maxillofacial Surgery, University of Toronto, Toronto, Ontario, Canada

SAVERIO CAPODIFERRO, DMD
Department of Interdisciplinary Medicine, University of Bari "Aldo Moro," Bari, Italy

BEHZAD CHESHMI, DDS
Professional Member, Maxillofacial Surgery and Implantology, Biomaterial Research Foundation, Tehran, Iran

TERPSITHEA CHRISTOU, DDS, MS, ABO
Assistant Professor and Clinical Director, School of Dentistry, The University of Alabama at Birmingham, Birmingham, Alabama, USA

NEOPHYTOS DEMETRIADES, MD, MSc
Oral and Maxillofacial Surgery, European University of Cyprus School of Medicine, Facial Plastic and Reconstructive Surgery, European University of Cyprus School of Medicine, Nicosia, Cyprus

TATAKIS DIMITRIS, DDS, PhD
Division of Periodontology, College of Dentistry, The Ohio State University, Columbus, Ohio, USA

MAZIAR SHAHZAD DOWLATSHAHI, DDS, MSc
Private Practice, Toronto, Ontario, Canada

HAMID REZA FALLAHI, DDS, OMFS
Oral and Maxillofacial Surgeon, Founder and Director, Maxillofacial Surgery and Implantology, Biomaterial Research Foundation, Tehran, Iran

ROBERT L. FLINT, DMD, MD
Associate Professor and Residency Program Director, Oral and Maxillofacial Surgery Department, University of Louisville, Louisville, Kentucky, USA

SHOHREH GHASEMI, DDS, Msc
Adjunct Assistant Professor, Department of Oral and Maxillofacial surgery, Augusta University, Augusta, Georgia, USA

PARASTOO JAFARI, DDS, MSc
Periodontist and Implantologist, Private Practice

MARTIN KASIR, MD
Worldwide Laser Institute, Dallas, Texas, USA

CHUNG HOW KAU, BDS, MScD, MBA, PhD, MOrth, FDSGlas, FDSEdin, FFDIre, FAMS(Ortho), FICD, FACD, ABO
Professor and Department Chair, School of Dentistry, The University of Alabama at Birmingham, Birmingham, Alabama, USA

RADA KAZAKOVA, DMD, PhD
Department of Prosthetic Dentistry, Faculty of Dental Medicine, Medical University – Plovdiv, Bulgaria

SEIED OMID KEYHAN, DDS, OMFS
Oral and Maxillofacial Surgeon, Founder and Director, Maxillofacial Surgery and Implantology, Biomaterial Research Foundation, Tehran, Iran; Co-Investigator, Department of Oral and Maxillofacial Surgery, College of Medicine, Jacksonville, Florida, USA

ARASH KHOJASTEH, MS, DMD, PhD
Professor, Department of Oral and Maxillofacial Surgery, School of Dentistry, Shahid Beheshti University of Medical Sciences, Tehran, Iran; Visiting Professor, Department of Health and Medical Sciences, University of Antwerp, Antwerp, Belgium

SEONG-GON KIM, DDS, PhD
Department of Oral and Maxillofacial Surgery, College of Dentistry, Gangneung-Wonju National University, Gangneung, Republic of Korea

JESSICA M. LATIMER, DDS
Department of Oral Medicine, Infection, and Immunity, Harvard School of Dental Medicine, Boston, Massachusetts, USA

EDWARD McLAREN, DMD
Private practice, Park City, Utah

FRANCESCO LUIGI MINTRONE, DMD
Department of Dentistry and Oral Maxillo Facial Surgery, University of Modena and Reggio Emilia, Modena, Italy

SADRA MOHAGHEGH, DMD
Research Assistant, Department of Oral and Maxillofacial Surgery, School of Dentistry, Shahid Beheshti University of Medical Sciences, Tehran, Iran

MARIO POLO, DMD, MS, FICD
Diplomate, American Board of Orthodontics; Private Practice, Orthodontics and Facial Esthetics, Assistant Professor (Ad Honorem), Department of Orthodontics, University of Puerto Rico School of Dental Medicine, San Juan, Puerto Rico, USA; Associate Editor, American Journal of Orthodontics & Dentofacial Orthopedics

ANDRÉ P. SAADOUN, DMD, MS
Diplomate, American Academy of Periodontology; Diplomate of the International Congress of Oral Implantologists; Private Practice limited to Esthetic Periodontics and Implant Surgery, Paris, France

AHMED SABBAH, DDS, PhD
Clinical Assistant Professor, Program Director, Advanced Education in General Dentistry Program, Department of Comprehensive Dentistry, University of Texas Health Science Center at San Antonio

POOYAN SADR-ESHKEVARI, DDS, MD
Resident Physician, Oral and Maxillofacial Surgery Department, University of Louisville, Louisville, Kentucky, USA

SHUBAM SHARMA, BDS, MPH
Orthodontic Resident, School of Dentistry, The University of Alabama at Birmingham, Birmingham, Alabama, USA

DIMITRIS N. TATAKIS, DDS, PhD, FICD
Diplomate, American Board of Periodontology; Professor and Director, Advanced Education Program, Division of Periodontology, Director for Global Initiatives, College of Dentistry, The Ohio State University, Columbus, Ohio, USA

PARISA YUSEFI, DDS, MS
Department of Prosthodontics, School of Dentistry, Isfahan University of Medical Sciences, Isfahan, Iran

CONTENTS

Preface   xiii

Behnam Bohluli, Shahrokh C. Bagheri, and Seied Omid Keyhan

Smile Analysis: Diagnosis and Treatment Planning   307

Ahmed Sabbah

Smile design is defined as the process of creating an esthetic smile based on scientific and artistic guidelines established through studies, perception, and cultural and racial standards that have been recognized over time. Smile design is a dynamic field with evolving trends that take into consideration: facial esthetics, lip dynamics, pink and white esthetics, and personality. Traditional smile design focused on the orodental complex. Modern smile designers must have a global understanding of the entire patient to design the perfect smile.

An Overview of Maxillofacial Approaches to Smile Design   343

Pooyan Sadr-Eshkevari, Robert L. Flint, and Brian Alpert

The oral and maxillofacial surgeon (OMS) has the knowledge and skills to make drastic skeletal changes in favor of a more cosmetic smile. OMS can also alter intraoral and extraoral soft tissues to make subtle or significant changes in facial cosmesis. This article provides an overview of the scope of the OMS in smile design. The authors provide a cursory review of pertinent gross and surgical facial anatomy, discuss the role of orthognathic surgery and rhinoplasty in smile cosmesis, and describe the fundamentals of common cosmetic procedures ranging from gingivoplasty to lip lift and lip augmentation and the use of neurotoxins.

Crown Lengthening Techniques and Modifications to Treat Excessive Gingival Display   361

Maziar Shahzad Dowlatshahi, Ghazal Anoosh, Jorge Alania, and
Jessica M. Latimer

Dental aesthetics are a fundamental treatment goal in dentistry, in which even minute deviations from the ideal may necessitate corrective treatment or constitute a suboptimal clinical outcome. A well-defined protocol that adheres to sound biological and surgical principles is necessary to harmoniously integrate the dental and periodontal components. This article reviews clinical and aesthetic guidelines based on these principles for clinical crown lengthening.

Lip Repositioning Techniques and Modifications   373

Dimitris N. Tatakis

A common etiology of excessive gingival display is hypermobile upper lip, which can be managed by non-surgical and surgical approaches. Among the surgical options, lip repositioning surgery is a relatively simple procedure with minimal complications. Since the original description of the technique almost 50 years ago, several minor and major modifications have been introduced. The available evidence indicates that, when applied to properly diagnosed cases, the technique is effective in reducing gingival display and results in improved smile esthetics and high patient satisfaction. This article reviews the various techniques and modifications and summarizes the reported outcomes of the procedure.

Orthognathic Surgery for Management of Gummy Smile   385

Arash Khojasteh and Sadra Mohaghegh

Excessive gingival show is mainly caused by hypermobility of the upper lip, altered passive eruption, gingival hyperplasia, and bony maxillary vertical excess. Orthognathic surgery is the optimal treatment option for patients with moderate and severe vertical maxillary excess. Surrounding anatomic structures and soft tissue changes such as alternation in the nasal morphology confine the amount of impaction. Therefore, Le Fort 1 may be performed in conjunction with horseshoe osteotomy or partial turbinectomy. The possible necessity of further mandibular orthognathic surgeries and chin repositioning has to be considered. No common major complication and long-term relapse have been reported for maxillary impaction.

Laser-Assisted Gingivectomy to Treat Gummy Smile   399

Saverio Capodiferro and Rada Kazakova

Excessive gingival display (EGD) is the extensive exposure of the gingiva during a smile. It is a common concern among patients, which may compromise the esthetic outcome of the dental treatment. Dental lasers demonstrate several advantages for soft tissue dental surgery compared with conventional surgical methods related to their technical characteristics. Owing to the excellent coagulation, especially of the surgical lasers, reduced to no need of anesthesia or suturing and faster healing, they demonstrate optimal clinical results. Nevertheless, good knowledge of laser–tissue interaction is required to obtain the best predictable results without gingival recession or bone tissue damage.

Botulinum Toxin and Smile Design   419

Mario Polo

Smiles with excessive gingival display exceeding 3 mm are considered unattractive. Excessive muscular contraction of lip elevator muscles is the etiology in most cases, and other factors, such as excessive vertical dimension of the maxilla and altered passive dental eruption resulting in the presence of excessive gingival tissue, account for the etiologic factors in others. Botulinum toxin type A (BTX-A) blocks muscular contraction by inhibiting the release of acetylcholine in muscles' endplates. The author has proven BTX-A to be an effective treatment alternative for the correction of these conditions affecting smile esthetics. This article explains how this is accomplished.

Lip Augmentation   431

Shohreh Ghasemi and Zahra Akbari

Just as priceless procedure of art and science needs the visual frame to bring out the subtle proportion to your face and bring out the best frame for the smile. Lip augmentation procedures with hyaluronic acid dermal fillers have become increasingly popular worldwide because full lips are often considered beautiful and youthful. The objective of a lip augmentation procedure is to create smooth lips with adequate volume and a natural appearance and not to be over corrected. Various techniques for lip augmentation have been used and described.

Lip Lift Techniques in Smile Design   443

Hamid Reza Fallahi, Seied Omid Keyhan, Behnam Bohluli, Behzad Cheshmi, and Parastoo Jafari

The lips are the main aesthetic component of the facial lower third and simultaneously a substantial element for an ideally perceived smile. One of the most accepted and common procedures that is widely used to enhance the shape and contours of the upper lip is the lip lift. With a careful treatment plan and a professional surgery, a lip lift can reliably be used for the reduction of the philtrum height, enlargement of the upper vermilion, improvement of the dental show, restoration of facial aesthetic proportions, and creation of an enchanting smile.

Contemporary Smile Design: An Orthodontic Perspective   459

Chung How Kau, Terpsithea Christou, and Shubam Sharma

Orthodontists play a vital role in the smile design of individuals. There are a variety of orthodontic goals and tooth movements that can be achieved to obtain the ideal smile that ultimately leads to the optimum esthetic outcomes. In this article, some methods and appliance systems to control and achieve the desired tooth movements are described and illustrated.

Smile Design: Mechanical Considerations   477

Marzieh Alikhasi, Parisa Yousefi, and Kelvin I. Afrashtehfar

Smile designing refers to the cosmetic and esthetic dental reconstruction that is visible during smiling. The use of modern digital tools requires adequate knowledge about the tooth shape and shade principles. Mechanical, biological, and psychological factors should be understood and tailor an individualized treatment accordingly to achieve pleasing esthetic outcomes. Dental therapy is becoming more appearance-driven, and thus, both patients and dental clinicians mainly emphasize on cosmetic dental and facial aspects of treatments.

Smile Management: A Discussion with the Masters   489

Behnam Bohluli, Seied Omid Keyhan, André P. Saadoun, Tatakis Dimitris, Edward McLaren, Francesco Luigi Mintrone, Neophytos Demetriades, Seong-Gon Kim, Shohreh Ghasemi, and Martin Kasir

Smile design is an ongoing challenge in both dentistry and facial cosmetics surgery. Herein, some very common smile design scenarios are shared with world known masters. Each case will be reviewed by cosmetic dentists, periodontists, dermatologists, and oral and maxillofacial surgeons. At the end, contributors will describe current advances and future prospects of this evolving field.

DENTAL CLINICS OF NORTH AMERICA

FORTHCOMING ISSUES

October 2022
Dental Biomaterials
Jack L. Ferracane, Luiz E. Bertassoni,
and Carmem S. Pfeifer, *Editors*

January 2023
Orofacial Pain Case Histories
with Literature Reviews
David A. Keith, Michael E. Schatman,
Ronald J. Kulich, and Steven J. Scrivani,
Editors

April 2023
Temporomandibular Disorders: The Current
Perspective
Davis C. Thomas and Steven R. Singer,
Editors

RECENT ISSUES

April 2022
Special Care Dentistry
Stephanie M. Munz, *Editor*

January 2022
Biologics and Biology-based Regenerative
Treatment Approaches in Periodontics
Alpdogan Kantarci, Andreas Stavropoulos,
and Anton Sculean, *Editors*

October 2021
Adolescent Oral Health
Deborah Studen-Pavlovich, *Editor*

SERIES OF RELATED INTEREST

Atlas of the Oral and Maxillofacial Surgery Clinics

Oral and Maxillofacial Surgery Clinics

THE CLINICS ARE AVAILABLE ONLINE!
Access your subscription at:
www.theclinics.com

Preface

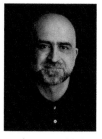 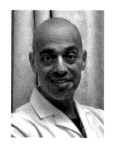 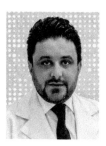

Behnam Bohluli,	Shahrokh C. Bagheri,	Seied Omid Keyhan,
DMD, FRCD(C)	DMD, MD, FACS, FICD	DDS, OMFS
	Editors	

Smile management has gradually evolved throughout several generations. The first documented attempts for smile management date back to the late 1970s when several sporadic reports showed how upper jaw surgery can correct the gummy smile. Thereafter, for a long time, smile management was limited to correction of the gummy smile patients with Le Fort osteotomy. Later, in 1982, Epker and his colleague published a landmark textbook that described etiology, diagnosis, and the treatment of the gummy smile by a team of orthodontists and oral and maxillofacial surgeons.[1] Though these pioneer works are still the mainstay in the treatment of structural gummy smiles, and though this surgery is currently done with minimum morbidity and downtime, many patients and practitioners have been looking for a more conservative approach.

Lip repositioning is one of the earliest endeavors to find a noninvasive way to manage the gummy smile. In 1979, two plastic surgeons, Litton and Fournier,[2] presented a simple approach to correct excessive gum show. In their approach, an elliptical piece of gum and lip is resected, and the upper lip is fixed to its new position. This technique has faded in an out several times in literature, and now it seems that lip repositioning is fully fledged in modern smile design with clear indications and techniques.

Use of botulinum toxin in smile improvement is an emerging concept that was first introduced by an orthodontist, Polo,[3] in 2004. Though the idea still has many challenging details, such as target muscles to be paralyzed, dosage, and number of injection sites, the idea is definitely supported by literature and now is a known off-label use of botulinum toxin in facial cosmetic medicine.

Lips are the last component of the smile that are commonly underestimated in smile design. Lip lift is a known cosmetic surgery that is done for both lip rejuvenation and cosmetics. Lip augmentation is the other growing trend that directly affects smile design.[4]

Teeth are the other determinant components of an ideal smile that have dramatically developed in last decades with few revolutionary concepts. Ackerman and Ackerman[5] are two orthodontists (2002) who used digital software to analyze and plan the smile design. This innovative work may be credited as the formal opening of digital era in dentistry. Edward McLaren in 2004 describes a practical approach to use photoshop

Dent Clin N Am 66 (2022) xiii–xiv
https://doi.org/10.1016/j.cden.2022.04.001
0011-8532/22/© 2022 Published by Elsevier Inc.

dental.theclinics.com

software for smile design. This simple innovation is another turning point in smile management that makes all the steps more predictable and reproducible. And finally, Christian Coachman and his colleagues[6] in 2017 introduced the digital smile design that is commonly known as a true revolution in smile management and probably in dentistry.

This issue of *Dental Clinics of North America* aims to present *New Horizons in Smile Design*. The editors of this issue believe that the multidisciplinary approach and digital technology are the backbone of the current and future smile design. Therefore, the main goal of this issue has been bridging all the above-mentioned islands in smile design and providing a real multidisciplinary reference for this challenging subject. Meanwhile, special attention has been given to digital smile concepts, which is fundamental to the most modern dental, surgical, and cosmetic approaches to smile design.

Behnam Bohluli, DMD, FRCD(C)
Departement of Oral and Maxillofacial Surgery
University of Toronto
Toronto, ON, Canada

Shahrokh C. Bagheri, DMD, MD, FACS, FICD
Georgia Oral &
Facial Reconstructive Surgery
Northside Hospital
Council of Scientific Affairs, ADA

Seied Omid Keyhan, DDS, OMFS
Maxillofacial Surgery & Implantology Biomaterial Research Foundation
Tehran, Iran

E-mail addresses:
bbohluli@yahoo.com (B. Bohluli)
sbagher@hotmail.com (S.C. Bagheri)
keyhanomid@ymail.com (S.O. Keyhan)

REFERENCES

1. Epker BN, Larry M. Dentofacial Deformities: Surgical-orthodontic Correction. Wolford Mosby 1980.
2. Litton C, Fournier P. Simple surgical correction of the gummy smile. Plast Reconstr Surg 1979;63(3):372-3.
3. Polo M. Botulinum toxin type A in the treatment of excessive gingival display. Am J Orthod Dentofacial Orthop 2005;127(2):214–8, quiz 261.
4. Ding A. The Ideal Lips: Lessons Learnt from the Literature. Aesthetic Plast Surg 2021;45(4):1520-30.
5. Ackerman MB, Ackerman JL. Smile analysis and design in the digital era. J Clin Orthod 2002;36(4):221-36.
6. Coachman C, Calamita MA, Sesma N. Dynamic documentation of the smile and the 2D/3D digital smile design process. Int J Periodontics Restorative Dent 2017;37(2):183–93. https://doi.org/10.11607/prd.2911. PMID: 2819615.

Smile Analysis
Diagnosis and Treatment Planning

Ahmed Sabbah, DDS, PhD

KEYWORDS

- Diastemas • Maxillary • Orthodontics • Smile • Smile Design
- Interdisciplinary Treatment Planning • Lip • Gingiva • Smile Arc • facial flow
- Airway • Global Diagnosis • FGTP • Digital Smile Design

INTRODUCTION
The Power of a Smile

"Even the simulation of an emotion tends to arouse it in our minds."[1] Charles Darwin was the first to explain the hidden power of a smile. In his Facial-Feedback hypothesis, he suggests that a smile has a systematically positive effect on the mind and body. A widely cited 30-year longitudinal study on the analysis of smile expression in women's college pictures revealed that women displaying positive emotions in pictures had favorable outcomes in their marriages and well-being and had more favorable personalities.[2] Another study found that people with new smiles altered by cosmetic dentistry were regarded as more attractive, intelligent, interesting, and wealthier.[3] The power of the smile is clearly exponential, and we are the architects of the new smile.

What Is Smile Design?

Smile design is defined as the process of creating an esthetic smile based on scientific and artistic guidelines established through studies, perception, and cultural and racial standards that have been recognized over time.[4] Smile design is a dynamic field with evolving trends that take into consideration: facial esthetics, lip dynamics, pink and white esthetics, and personality. Traditional smile design focused on the orodental complex. Modern smile designers must have a global understanding of the entire patient to design the perfect smile. Subjectivity is fundamental when it comes to smile design. Purely scientific smiles are generic, symmetric, and seem fake. Copying and pasting the same smile using the same tooth library and gingival esthetics for each patient results in an unesthetic result. No 2 smiles are identical, and each smile must take on an identity of its own based on the guidelines outlined later. In the era of social media, it is popular for dentists to showcase artificial smiles. What sets a beautiful smile apart is the integration of organic guidelines to achieve "perfect" results. In essence, embracing nature and its imperfections is the next level of smile design (**Fig. 1**).

Advanced Education in General Dentistry Program, Department of Comprehensive Dentistry, University of Texas Health Science Center at San Antonio, 8210 Floyd Curl Drive San Antonio, TX 78229, USA
E-mail address: SABBAH@uthscsa.edu

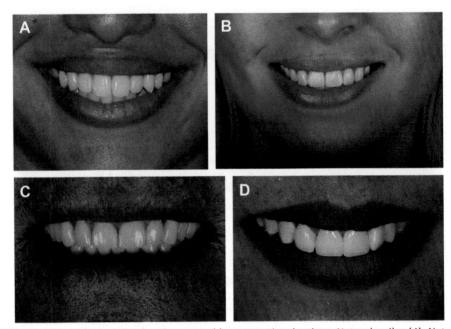

Fig. 1. Natural and artificial smiles created by restorative dentistry. Natural smiles (*A*). Natural smile (*B*). Artificial smiles (*C*). Artificial smile (*D*).

Global Components of the Smile

In this section, the authors discuss the fundamentals of smile analysis and the parameters to design the most esthetic smile. The term *Ideal smile* has been used in the literature; however, as discussed one can argue that no smile is ideal and that "Beauty is in the eye of the beholder."[4] As such no smile design is successful without the comprehensive involvement of the patient. Therefore, the first step in smile design is *patient communication*. In the era of digital dentistry, several applications and software exist that can facilitate discussions with patients and understanding of expectations and possibilities.

Three smile types have been shown in the literature: commissure smile (Mona Lisa smile), social smile (cuspid smile), and spontaneous smile (complex smile)[5] (**Fig. 2**). *Smile design should be performed on the patient's spontaneous smile, as it depicts true emotions*. The social smile is usually used to disguise negative aspects of their

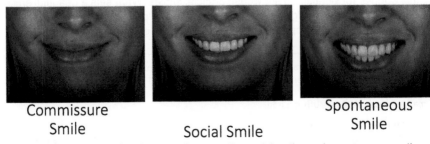

Commissure
Smile

Social Smile

Spontaneous
Smile

Fig. 2. Different types of smile: commissure smile, social smile, and spontaneous smile.

smile and should not be used. It is challenging to get a patient in a dental chair to reproduce a spontaneous smile. Therefore, the recommendation is to film the patient in a nontreatment room with a relaxed ambiance. Several frames are cropped from the video to provide dynamic data of the patient's smile.[6] Failure to recognize the spontaneous smile can lead to incorrect diagnosis and catastrophic failure.

The four building blocks of the modern esthetic smile

1. Facial esthetics: in this section, the authors discuss determinants of facial esthetics (**Fig. 3**). All measurements are made in repose and natural head position. Repose is defined as a rest position with the teeth and lips slightly apart.[7] Natural head position is defined as a reproducible position of the head in an upright posture with the eyes focused on a point at eye level.[8]
   a. Facial view
      i. *Facial proportions:* the rule of thirds divides the face into 3 sections (**Fig. 4**). The heights and ratio of the middle to lower third in repose play a significant role in smile esthetics and diagnosis. The ideal ratio of the middle:lower third is 1:1. A longer lower third is diagnosed as vertical maxillary excess (VME) and can result in a gummy smile.[7] A shorter lower third may indicate a reduced occlusal vertical dimension (OVD).
      ii. *Reference lines:* the 3 reference lines used in modern smile design in a frontal view are the *interpupillary line (IPL), the commissural line (CL), and the facial flow* (**Fig. 5**).[9] The IPL is defined as a straight line that passes through the pupils and is used to determine the transverse position of the maxillary occlusal plane. The CL is determined by a straight line drawn between the right and left lip commissure.[9] Parallelism between the IPL and CL results in facial harmony. A recent report analyzed top celebrity smiles and found that the most esthetic smiles were when the IPL, CL, and occlusal plane were all parallel.[10]

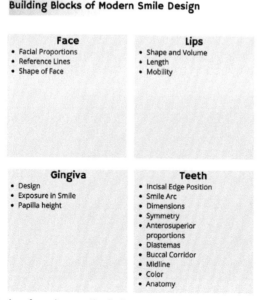

Fig. 3. Building blocks of modern smile design.

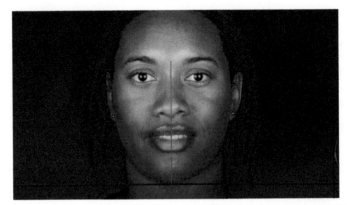

Fig. 4. Facial proportions: middle to lower third ideally is 1:1. A longer lower third is diagnosed as VME (patient consent). This patient's middle third measures at 64 mm and lower third is 74 mm.

In situations where there is a lack of parallelism between the IPL and CL, laypeople preferred the occlusal plane to be parallel with the CL.[11] The facial midline is a straight line drawn through the glabella, the tip of the nose, philtrum, and the tip of the chin.[9] More recently, emphasis has been given to the *facial flow* concept that states that due to the natural asymmetry of the human face, it is impossible to define a straight line as the midline. Rather, a curved line connecting facial landmarks is more acceptable.[12] The relationship of the dental midline with the facial flow is discussed later in this article.

  b. Profile view

    i. Reference lines (**Fig. 6**)

      1. *The Frankfort horizontal*, which is defined as a straight line from the highest point on the margin of the auditory meatus to the lowest point of the orbit, should be parallel to the horizon when the patient is in NHP.[13]

      2. *Camper's plane or Ala-Tragus line*, which is a line running from the inferior border of the ala to the superior border of the tragus of the ear, determines the maxillary occlusal plane.[13,14] Different systems have shown reliability in reproducing the maxillary occlusal plane, such as the Kois Dento-

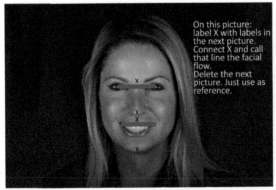

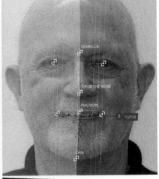

Fig. 5. Facial reference lines: the interpupillary line, the commissural line, and the facial flow line as shown in the figure.

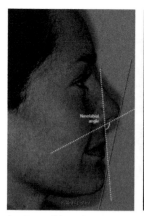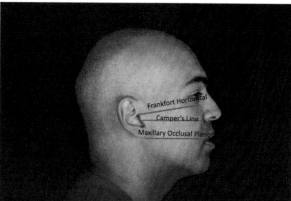

Fig. 6. Profile reference lines. The Frankfort horizontal, Camper line, nasiolabial angle, and E-Line are all important in smile design. (*From* Levine JB, Finkel S. Smile Design Integrating Esthetics and Function. Vol Volume Two. (Levine JB, ed.). ELSEVIER; 2016.)

Facial Analyzer, virtual face-bows, and the Behrend system that relies on the use of photographs to determine tooth position and is the prototype of Digital Smile Design (DSD).[15]

3. *Nasolabial angle:* this is an angle created at the subnasale by the intersection of a tangent to the base of the nose with a tangent to the outer edge of the upper lip.[9] In individuals with normal profile the angle is between 90° and 95° in men and 95° to 115° in women. Smaller angles indicate a prominent maxilla and excessive lip support. Less dominant restorations are recommended in these situations.[9]

4. *Ricketts E-plane:* a line drawn from the tip of the nose to the chin. In most races, the upper lip is about 2 to 4 mm posterior to the line, whereas the lower lip is 0 to 2 mm posterior in a normal profile. In a concave profile (angle class III malocclusion), the lower lip is in front of the line. The maxillary centrals can be made more dominant to get closer to the E-line. Conversely, in a convex patient (angle class II malocclusion), the lower lip is more than 2 mm behind the line and the maxillary centrals should be less dominant.[7,16]

c. *Facial shapes:* "The law of harmony" suggested a correlation between facial shape and contours of upper permanent incisors. The facial shapes described are oval, triangle, and square.[17] More recently, a correlation between facial shape, personality, and tooth shapes has been proposed in what is called Visual Identity of a Smile (VIS).[18]

2. Lip esthetics

a. *Lip shape and volume:* lips are classified as thin, medium, or thick. Voluminous lips are seen as more attractive in women with the lower lip closer to the E-line (**Fig. 7**).[19] Slightly protruding inverted upper lips have been shown to convey youth and attractiveness.[20] In men less prominent lips are a sign of masculinity and social dominance.[21] With voluminous lips being the current standard of beauty, care should be taken when retroclining maxillary incisors to avoid negative impacts on lip volume.[20]

b. *Lip length* (**Fig. 8**): the upper lip is measured from the base of the nose to the inferior border of the upper lip. A normal upper lip measures 20 mm to

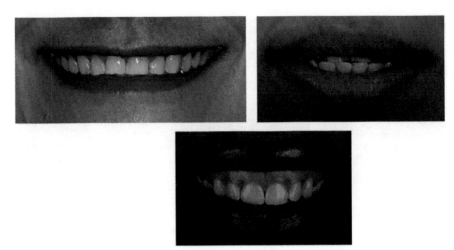

Fig. 7. Different types of lips: thin, medium, and thick.

22.0 mm in women and 22 mm to 24 mm in men.[22] A long upper lip decreases incisal display, resulting in a less esthetic smile. Lip lifting is a technique that can be used to unveil maxillary incisors.[20] Conversely, a short upper lip results in excessive incisal display and a possible gummy smile and can be treated by Botox.[7]

c. *Lip mobility* **Fig. 9**: upper lip mobility is defined as the amount of lip movement in a full smile; this can be measured by subtracting incisal exposure at rest from dentogingival exposure during a spontaneous smile or by subtracting lip length in a spontaneous smile from lip length in repose.[22] Normal lip mobility is 6 to 8 mm.[7] A hypermobile lip can be treated using Botox.

d. *Lower lip*: the role of the lower lip in smile esthetics has not been analyzed as comprehensively even though the lower lip creates the smile frame. The current standard of beauty is a voluminous lower lip. Furthermore, the maxillary incisal edge should touch the lower lip in a social smile; however, a 0.5 mm gap was still considered esthetic.[23] The smile index is defined as the intercommisural width divided by the interlabial gap during a smile (**Fig. 10**).[24] Generally, an

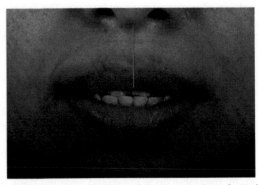

Fig. 8. A. Lip length. Measured from the base of the nose to the inferior border of the upper lip.

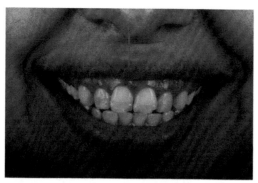

Fig. 9. Lip mobility. Length of blue line to red line = 9 mm. Hypermobile. Lip resulting in excessive gingival display.

esthetic smile index is greater than 5.0 and less than 7.5.[25] A spontaneous smile with interocclusal space will generally have a greater smile index than a posed smile. A smile index greater than 7.5 indicates the aging of a smile due to the greater width and the smaller interlabial gap. If the upper lip and maxillary occlusal planes are in the ideal position, the reduced interlabial gap is due to the higher position of the lower lip position, which could be due to the reduced OVD.

3. *Gingival esthetics*: gingival architecture is fundamental to smile design. Color, stippling, and biotype are essential components of pink esthetics.
   a. *Gingival design:* as discussed by Fradeani, the gingival margin should maintain parallelism with the occlusal plane and horizontal references such as the IPL and CL (**Fig. 11**).[9] Furthermore, the gingival margin should maintain the proper curvature to match incisal edges and the smile arc. Soft tissue grafting and crown lengthening are periodontal procedures used to achieve harmonious gingival margins. The classic gingival design is where the canines and central incisor gingival margin falls on the same line with the laterals slightly coronal (1–2 mm).[5] Variations exist such as the modified gingival designed where the centrals and laterals are on the same line. The classic literature has focused on the anterior 6; however, with the focus on wider smiles, the posterior teeth gingival margins should be taken into consideration. Crawford and colleagues[26] suggested the esthetic zone for posterior teeth, which is defined as a tangent

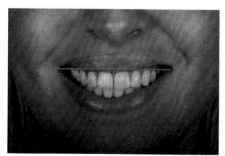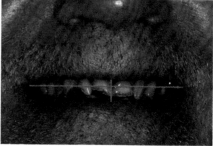

Fig. 10. Smile index = intercommisural width/interlabial gap. The esthetic range is 5 to 7.5. A greater smile index could be related to a smaller interlabial gap due to a collapsed OVD.

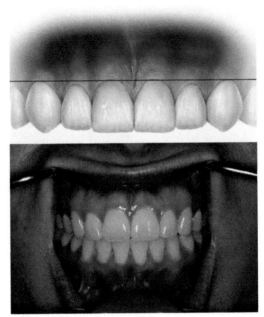

Fig. 11. Ideal gingival design. (1) Canine sand centrals on a straight line; (2) laterals slightly incisal to the line. Gingival margin follows smile arc. (*From* Levine JB, Finkel S. Smile Design Integrating Esthetics and Function. Vol Volume Two. (Levine JB, ed.). ELSEVIER; 2016.)

from the canine margin to the lower border of the upper lip superior to the first molar. An acceptable range for the premolars is 2 mm apical to the line and 1 mm for molars. Further studies are needed to evaluate posterior teeth esthetics as the demand for wider smiles increases. The gingival zenith is defined as the most apical point of the gingival margin. Traditionally, the zenith is located slightly distal to the midline of the centrals and in the center for laterals and canines.[27]

  b. *Gingival exposure:* Robbins and colleagues[7] suggested that gingival display more than 2 mm in a high smile is regarded as excessive. In the spontaneous smile, Machado and colleagues[5] suggested that 3 mm is the threshold for a gummy smile. Therefore we suggest that gingival exposure of more than 2 to 3 mm is regarded as excessive (**Fig. 12**). Treatment of a gummy smile depends on the *Global Diagnosis system* discussed later in this article.

  c. *Papillary height:* Hochman and colleagues[28] reported that the length of the papilla was 40% the length of the tooth from the zenith to the incisal edge. Furthermore, they reported that 87% of patients with low smiles displayed papilla. Therefore, when designing smiles of patients with low smiles, it is crucial to maintain the papillary display.[28] Long contacts with no papilla are regarded as unesthetic and should be avoided. Tooth and restoration shapes play an important role in papilla height. Triangular and oval-shaped restorations have shorter contacts and longer papilla. If the height from the base of the contact to the crest of the bone is more than 5 mm then a longer contact or more square restoration is necessary to avoid the formation of a black triangle.[29]

4. *Dental esthetics:* in this section, the authors discuss different specifics of white esthetics that need to be taken into consideration during smile design.

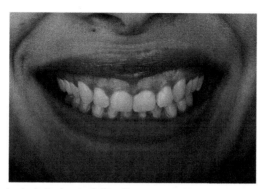

Fig. 12. Excessive gingival display in full smile.

a. *Incisal edge position:* this is the most important factor in determining tooth position in smile design. Maxillary central incisal edge is determined in repose and full smile. In repose, if lip length is normal, the incisal edge display is 3 to 4 mm in women and 1 to 2 mm in men (**Fig. 13**).[30] More incisal display indicates a more youthful and attractive smile. In full smile, Gaikwad and colleagues[23,31] reported that the best esthetic result is when the maxillary centrals contacted the lower lip even though 0.5 mm distance between the incisal edge and the lower lip was still considered esthetic. Moreover, Pound reported that in an E-Smile (spontaneous) the maxillary centrals should occupy between 50% and 80% of the interlabial distance.[32] The F sounds are also used to determine the incisal edge position. During gentle pronunciation of the F sounds, the incisal edge should touch the wet/dry border of the lower lip.[16]

b. *Smile Arc:* smile arc refers to the position of the maxillary incisors in a vertical position. Profitt and colleagues[33] reported that the smile arc is the most important factor of the smile. Smile arc is classified into 3 categories: convex/positive, straight/plane, or inverted/reverse (**Fig. 14**). The positive smile is the most esthetic and is defined as when the maxillary incisal edges cradle the lower lip. Al Johany and colleagues[34] found that positive smiles were seen in 78% of celebrity smiles. In a positive smile, the incisal edge of the maxillary central is more incisal than the canines. Furthermore, there is a 0.5 to 1 mm step between the incisal edge of the maxillary centrals and the laterals in men and 1.0 to 1.5 mm step in women.[5] This ensures the dominance of the maxillary centrals. To create a less dominant smile, the clinician can decrease the maxillary-lateral incisal edge step and position the maxillary central incisal edge at the same level as the canine edge.

c. *Maxillary central dimensions and symmetry:* once the vertical position of the maxillary centrals is established, the length and the width need to be determined. The range for width:height ratio of the maxillary centrals is 75% to 85%.[35] Slender teeth are more common in women, whereas male teeth are closer to 85%. Any ratio greater than 85% is regarded as unesthetic. The esthetic guide for hard tissue developed by Chu and colleagues[36] uses mathematical formulas to calculate the width and height of maxillary and mandibular anteriors as well as intratooth relationships. If the width of the central is X, the lateral is X-2, whereas the canine is X-1. The height can then be calculated by dividing by 0.78 (dentist preferred W/H ratio) (**Fig. 15**). Based on this formula: the width of the mandibular central = X-3 and the average dimensions of the

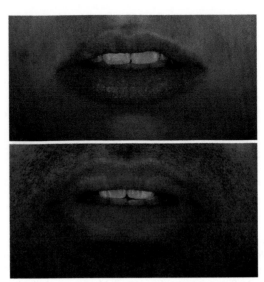

Fig. 13. Incisal edge position in repose. 3 to 4 mm in women and 1 to 2 mm in men.

centrals are 8.5 mm wide and 11 mm long. Gender and face size play a major role in teeth dimensions.[36] Natural smiles have a degree of asymmetry; however, symmetry was found to be most crucial for the maxillary central incisors. Asymmetry was less noticeable further from the midline.[37]

d. *Proportions between anterosuperior teeth:* the intertooth relationship between the maxillary anteriors has been studied extensively through the years. Levin proposed the golden ratio in 1978, which suggested that in the facial view the width of the laterals is 62% the width of the centrals and that the width of the canines is 62% the width of the laterals.[38] The golden proportion was found to not exist in nature and was regarded as unesthetic in several studies due to the narrowing of the smile.[39] With the emphasis on wider smiles in modern smile design, other proportions are regarded as more esthetic. The recurring esthetic dental (RED) proportion has been proposed by Ward and colleagues[40] as a model for modern smile design. RED proportion ranges from 62% to 80% and differs based on the desired length of teeth and height and gender of the patient. For shorter teeth, the 80% RED proportion was found to be the most esthetic, whereas for longer teeth the 62% RED (Golden) was ideal (**Fig. 16**).

e. *Presence of diastemas:* in general, all anterior diastemas should be closed unless requested by the patient. An untreated maxillary median diastema (MMD) of more than 0.5 mm was regarded as less esthetic[41] Moreover, MMD of more than 4 mm is recommended to be restored by an interdisciplinary approach of orthodontics and restorations.[41] In these cases the use of restorative alone results in abnormal tooth shape that does not follow the W/H ratio of 78%. Recently, Bioclear has been marketed as a solution for diastema closures. It is the authors' opinion that Bioclear results in W/H ratio greater than 78%, which produces an unesthetic smile with square teeth, long contacts, and papillary height less than 40%.

f. *Buccal corridors:* this is defined as the dark space between the buccal of the maxillary teeth and the labial commissure during smiling. Buccal corridors can be classified as narrow, intermediate, or wide.[5] The effect of the buccal

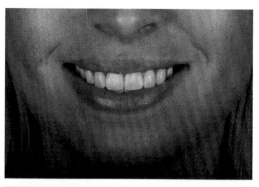

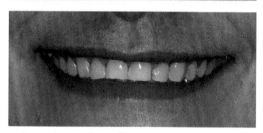

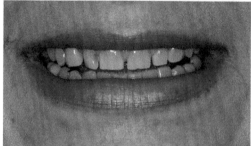

Fig. 14. Positive, straight, and negative smiles.

corridor on smile esthetics has been controversial, with some studies reporting that laypeople did not notice a difference, whereas other studies reported that an intermediate buccal corridor is more esthetic.[42] Furthermore, a recent study analyzing celebrity smiles found that only 22% of celebrity smiles had a wider

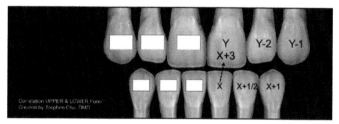

Fig. 15. Intratooth dimensions as proposed by Chu. (*From* German DS, Chu SJ, Furlong ML, Patel A. Simplifying optimal tooth-size calculations and communications between practitioners. Am J Orthod Dentofac. 2016;150(6):1051-1055. https://doi.org/10.1016/j.ajodo.2016.04.031.)

Different RED Proportions
(Central Incisor 78% w/l ratio)   Tooth Length

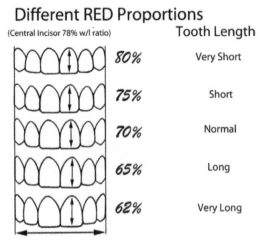

80%	Very Short
75%	Short
70%	Normal
65%	Long
62%	Very Long

Fig. 16. Different RED proportions for anterior teeth ratios. (*From* Ward DH. Proportional Smile Design. Dent Clin N Am. 2015;59(3):623-638. https://doi.org/10.1016/j.cden.2015.03.006.)

corridor.[43] A wide buccal corridor can be treated by camouflaging the space with restorative dentistry; however, a wider corridor usually indicates a narrow arch. With the current emphasis on airway in treatment planning, the ideal treatment modality should be maxillary expansion to position the teeth in the correct transverse position.[7]

g. *Midline position and angulation:* the position of the *maxillary midline* plays a controversial role in smile esthetics. Classic literature indicates that a midline shift of 3 to 4 mm was not recognized by laypeople.[44] In these studies, however, the face was not included, which undermines the importance of the face in smile design. More contemporary literature reports that a midline deviation of greater than 2 mm was regarded as unesthetic.[45] In addition, 48.8% of celebrity smiles had a midline deviation, which underscores that minimal deviation is not noticeable and should not alter the treatment plan to unnecessarily correct the maxillary midline.[43] Although the midline changes are not as noticeable, classic literature suggested that *angulation of the midline* had a more pronounced effect on smile esthetics. A cant of 2.0 mm in the midline was readily noticed by laypeople and resulted in an unesthetic smile.[44] More recently, the concept of *facial flow* has suggested that canting or shifting of the midline is acceptable if it follows the facial flow (**Fig. 17**). The direction that the facial flow points toward is called the green side. Angulation of the midline or shifting toward the green side is less noticeable, resulting in a blended-in effect. If the midline is shifted or canted toward the opposite direction (red side), greater visual tension occurs, resulting in an unesthetic smile.[12]

h. Tooth color and anatomy
   i. *Color:* studies have shown that brighter tooth shade significantly increased the attractiveness of a smile. Moreover, it was reported that women preferred lighter shades than men. Therefore, the current recommendation is to whiten teeth to a lighter shade before cosmetic procedures.[46] Furthermore, biomimetic dentistry advocates the use of minimally invasive restorations such as contact lens veneers with greater translucency, thus the stump shade would have greater effects on the final shade of the smile.

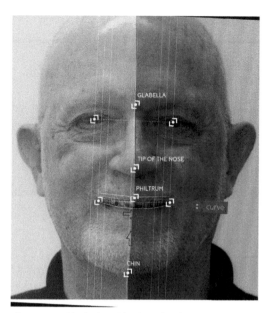

Fig. 17. Facial flow: the green side is the side that the dental midline can "flow" toward. A midline shift toward the red side is more noticeable.

ii. *Anatomy:* several anatomic components affect the shape of the smile (**Fig. 18**):[16]

1. Line angles: these give the general outline of the teeth and control the width. Altering the line angles can make a tooth look wider or narrower.
2. Height of contour: located distal to the midline in the gingival third. Anterior maxillary teeth have 3 planes.
3. Contacts: contact areas start at 40% at the midline and decrease distally. Contact points move more apically as in a distal direction.
4. Incisal embrasures: incisal embrasures increase gradually as we move distally starting at 20% of the tooth height at the midline to 35% at the distal of the canines.
5. Incisal edge: incisal edge anatomy and translucency are essential in creating a more natural smile. Younger patients have more defined incisal edges with mamelons. The opalescence that is seen at the incisal edge must be created in restorations to avoid the artificial look.
6. Texture: microtexture: these are developmental grooves that are found in younger teeth and usually run horizontally. Macrotexture refers to lobes that divide the facial surface of teeth into distinct concavities and convexities.[9]
7. Tooth shape: different concepts have been proposed to aid in the selection of tooth shapes and forms. Leon Williams proposed that the shape of the maxillary anteriors should match the face form. The 3 proposed shapes were square, triangular, and ovoid.[47] Contemporary teeth selection has focused on incorporating a patient's personal identity and facial features to create a more personalized smile.[18] Gurel and colleagues created the VIS, which developed an association between esthetics, function, artistic visual language, facial recognition, and personality typology to develop 4 smile design types outlined as follows:

Building blocks of modern smile design

Face	Lips
• Facial proportions • Reference lines • Shape of face	• Shape and volume • Length • Mobility
Gingiva	Teeth
• Design • Exposure in smile • Papilla height	• Incisal edge position • Smile arc • Dimensions • Symmetry • Anterosuperior proportions • Diastemas • Buccal corridor • Midline • Color • Anatomy

Fig. 18. Teeth anatomy fundamentals in modern smile design. (*From* Levine JB, Finkel S. Smile Design Integrating Esthetics and Function. Vol Volume Two. (Levine JB, ed.). ELSEVIER; 2016.)

  a. Strong: composed of mainly rectangular shapes, strong dominance
  b. Dynamic: triangular shapes, standard dominance
  c. Delicate: oval shapes, medium dominance.
  d. Calm or stable: smoothly rounded square with weak dominance
8. Teeth library: historically, the anatomy of restorations depended on the laboratory technician fabricating the case and their comfort level. Digital dentistry has opened the possibility for infinite libraries, shapes, and molds of teeth. In addition, patients can select and visualize a tooth library before fabrication; this is one of the main principles of DSD. In addition, digital dentistry allows us to "copy" natural libraries from one patient and "paste" them into another. This copy-paste concept was developed by Dr Christian Coahcman and emphasizes the use of natural teeth library to create a natural-looking smile, rather than using artificial libraries.

Clinical tip: all the following lead to aging of the smile and should be avoided during smile design[18]:

- Flattened incisal edges
- Smaller incisal embrasures
- Smoother facial texture
- Prominent mandibular display
- Increase chroma
- Anterior splaying

Contemporary Treatment Planning and Smile Design

So far, we have focused on the fundamentals of smile design. As suggested in the previous section, smile design is interdisciplinary. A practitioner who just focuses on esthetics without an understanding of airway, function, structure, and biology will always fail in treating most smile design cases. Patients who report for smile makeovers usually have complicated cause that has resulted in the unesthetic outcome presented.

Therefore, the modern smile design team should consist of general practitioners and specialists with interdisciplinary knowledge.

Several interdisciplinary treatment planning concepts have been developed over the years. Dr Roblee proposed the *interdisciplinary dentofacial therapy (IDT) model*.[48] Dr Roblee defines *IDT* as a synergist relationship "between" specialties rather than each specialty acting independently (multidisciplinary). The IDT model has evolved to the more contemporary model called mature IDT. Mature IDT focuses on an evidence-based approach with common goals and cloud-based communication. Communication had been the biggest challenge when dealing with these cases. The development of DSD and asynchronous communication by Dr Christian Coachman has revolutionized the treatment of these interdisciplinary cases.[49]

Another interdisciplinary treatment planning concept is the *facially generated treatment planning (FGTP)* approach proposed by Dr Frank Spear and Dr John Kois.[50] Traditional treatment planning focused on collecting data and findings through a comprehensive diagnostic approach with casts, radiographs, and a clinical examination to develop a treatment plan; this is an "inside-out" approach, starting with the biology, structure, function, and then esthetics of the teeth. As a result, the esthetic result was frequently compromised, as the end result could not be visualized ahead of time. Think about trying to put pieces of a puzzle together without knowing what the outcome should look like. Furthermore, the esthetic result relied primarily on the orodental complex without much attention to the face.

FACIALLY GENERATED TREATMENT PLANNING

The Great Pyramids of Giza are some of the wonders of the world that took 30 years each to build. Imagine the ancient Egyptians inspecting the structure of each block and stacking them one by one without having an end goal. Thirty years later they decide they did not like the final result. That is how inside-out treatment planning works (**Fig. 19**). The ancient Egyptians used an "outside-in" approach, where they visualized an end result, then reverse-engineer the construction. Frank Spear and John Kois were the first to adopt this "outside-in" approach to treatment planning.[50] The logic stemmed from the popular saying by Dr Peter Dawson: "If you know where are and know where you want to go, getting there is easy."[16] In essence, you need to know what the puzzle looks like before putting the pieces together. FGTP starts with the end in mind with emphasis on facial and dental *E*sthetics followed by *F*unction, *S*tructure, and *B*iology (EFSB system).[51] More recently, *A*irway has been added to the equation, where airway has become the first step in FGTP (AEFSB system) (**Fig. 20**). Instead of expanding the smile with veneers and camouflaging a constricted maxilla, expanding the airway with orthodontics would result in ideal esthetics while addressing airway issues resulting in a healthier outcome.[52] Linking esthetics to health emphasizes the newly discovered importance of ideal smile design in achieving overall health.

- *Airway phase:* this starts with the examination of the airway before deciding on the position of the teeth. The first step is a sleep questionnaire such as the Epworth Sleeping Scale (ESS), Berlin, or the Wisconsin sleep questionnaire.[53] A proper examination is needed that includes body mass index, craniofacial morphology, tongue, and pharyngeal size, palatine tonsils, and teeth wear patterns. Once airway involvement is suspected, several screening tools are recommended by Dr Jeff Rouse, such as high-resolution pulse oximetry (HRPO) for 2 to 3 days, which measures oxygen desaturation and pulse rate changes. If apnea is suspected, the patient is referred to a physician to diagnose sleep apnea. Several

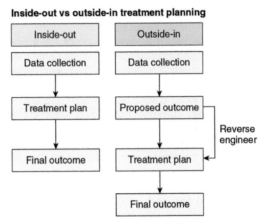

Fig. 19. Inside-out treatment planning versus outside in treatment planning.

treatment interventions are available to expand the airway as part of interdisciplinary treatment, such as surgically facilitated orthodontic therapy, miniscrew-assisted palatal expansion, or orthognathic surgery. These interventions lead to changes in teeth position and affect the smile frame. As a result, this model suggests that it is important to rule out airway issues before smile design.

- *Esthetic phase:* this phase consists of 8 steps based on the guidelines discussed earlier in this article:
  - *Central incisal edge position:* determine the position of the incisal edge in full smile and repose in a vertical position.
  - *Maxillary incisor inclination:* determine the labial inclination of the maxillary incisors.
  - *Maxillary occlusal plane:* determine the position of the rest of the maxillary teeth relative to esthetics.
  - *Gingival levels*: determine ideal gingival levels using the width and length proportions of each tooth and gingival displays as a guide.
  - *Mandibular incisor edge position*: determine the position of the mandibular incisor edge relative to the maxillary arch.
  - *Mandibular incisor occlusal relationship*: set the mandibular incisal edge against the lingual of the maxillary incisors; this determines the OVD.
  - *Mandibular occlusal plane:* the remaining mandibular teeth are set at the established OVD in the intercuspal position.
  - *Mandibular Gingival Levels:* Determine the position of the mandibular gingiva relative to appropriate tooth dimensions.
- *Functional phase:* the goal of this phase is to integrate the esthetic analysis with a functional occlusion. This phase consists of 3 steps:
  - *Joint signs and symptoms:* evaluation of the temporomandibular joint (TMJ) function and movement.
  - *Muscle pain and tenderness:* evaluation of muscles for signs of tenderness and pain.
  - *Dental signs and symptoms:* evaluation of signs of wear, fractures, sensitivity, and cracks.
- *Structural phase:* during this phase, the clinician determines the following:
  - Teeth that require treatment

AEFSB system in FGTP (Frank Spear)

Airway

- Sleep questionnaire
- Intraoral and extraoral exam
- Seattle protocol

Esthetics

- Central incisal edge
- Maxillary incisor inclination
- Maxillary occlusal plane
- Ideal gingival levels
- Mandibular incisal edge
- Mandibular incisal occlusal relationship
- Mandibular occlusal plane
- Mandibular gingival levels

Function

- Joint signs and symptoms
- Muscle pain and tenderness
- Dental signs and symptoms

Structure

- Teeth requiring treatment
- Teeth with inadequate struture to restore
- Teeth that will be removed
- Missing teeth that will be replaced
- Tooth replacement concerns

Biology

- Endodontics
- Periodontics
- Oral surgery required

Fig. 20. AEFSB system in facially generated treatment planning.

- Teeth with inadequate structure to restore
- Teeth that will be removed
- Missing teeth that will be replaced
- Tooth replacement concerns
- *Biological phase*: At the biological phase, the clinician takes into consideration endodontic therapy and periodontal care and oral surgery. The 3 steps for this phase are as follows:
  - Endodontics
  - Periodontics
  - Oral surgery.

GLOBAL DIAGNOSIS

In 2016 Robbins and Rouse established a model to address gingival display[7]. They concluded that even though the incisal edge position generated by FGTP was ideal, the final result may be unsatisfactory in some cases due to excessive gingival display. They developed the *Global Diagnosis* approach that focuses on the "gummy smile."[7] The 4, 5, 6 concept states that there are *(4) global diagnoses* for interdisciplinary treatment planning, *(5) core questions* to determine the diagnosis, and *(6) treatment options* (**Fig. 21**).

- The 4 global diagnoses:
  1. *Upper lip*: short/long or hypermobile/hypomobile
  2. *Clinical crowns:*
     - Short: microdontia, incisal wear or altered passive eruption
     - Long: recession
  3. Dentoalveolar extrusion (DAE)
  4. Skeletal discrepancy: vertical maxillary excess, vertical maxillary deficiency, angle class II or class III malocclusion
- *The 5 core questions:*[7]
  1. "What are the facial proportions?"
  - Normal middle:lower face is 1:1
  2. "What are the length and mobility of the upper lip?"
  - Normal lip length: 20 to 22 mm in women and 22 to 24 mm in men.
  - Normal lip mobility during smile: 6 to 8 mm in full smile.
  3. "What is the relationship between gingiva levels and the horizon?"
  - Straight line from canine to canine with centrals on the line and laterals 1 to 2 mm below the line
  4. "What is the length of maxillary central incisors?"
  - 10 to 11 mm
  5. "Is the cementoenamel junction (CEJ) palpable in the sulcus?"
  - CEJ should be detected in the sulcus

Once the dentist answers the 5 core questions, a Global Diagnosis can be made. In this section, *all 5 cores questions are assumed normal except for the one discussed.* It is possible that several variables can be affected in which case several Global Diagnoses would be considered.

1. *Vertical maxillary excess:* the patient has a longer lower face compared with the middle third. If the patient has a shorter lower face compared with the middle third, the diagnosis is *vertical maxillary deficiency.*
2. *Short upper lip*: the patient's lip is shorter in length than the standards discussed earlier. *Long upper lip*: the patient's lip is longer than the standards shown earlier (**Fig. 22**).
3. *Hypermobile upper lip:* the patient's lip moves more than 6 to 8 mm in full smile. If the patient's lip does not move 6 to 8 mm in full animation then the diagnosis is *hypomobile upper lip*
4. *Dentoalveolar extrusion:* in this case, the patient's gingiva is concave when drawing a line from canine to canine. The maxillary central incisors do not fall on the straight line. All other variables are normal, including palpation of the CEJ (**Fig. 23**).
5. *Microdontia:* the patient has smaller teeth than the norms discussed earlier. The CEJ is palpable, and there is no wear.
6. *Incisal attrition:* the patient has short teeth, CEJ is palpable, and there is incisal edge wear.
7. *Altered passive eruption:* the patient has short teeth, CEJ cannot be detected in the sulcus, and usually there is no wear on the incisal edge (**Fig. 24**).
8. *Recession:* the patient's teeth are long, and the CEJ is visible

Global diagnosis (Robbins and Rouse)	
4 Global diagnoses	**5 Core questions**

• Upper lip
  ◦ Short/long
  ◦ Hypermobile/hypomobile
• Clinical crowns
  ◦ Short microdontla, Incisal wear, APE
  ◦ Long
• Dentoalveolar extrusion
• Skeletal discrepancy: VME, VMD, class II, class III malocclusion
	1. Facial proportions?
	2. Length and mobility of upper lip?
	3. Gingival level VS horizon?
	4. Length of maxillary centrals?
	5. CEJ location?

6 Treatment Options	

• Orthognathic surgery
  ◦ Diagnosis VME. VMD. class II or III malocclusion
• Plastic surgery:
  ◦ Diagnosis short/long upper lip, hypermobile/hypomobile upper lip
• Orthodontics:
  ◦ Diagnosis: dentoalveolar extrusion
  ◦ Class II or III malocclusion
	• Restorations:
	  ◦ Diagnosis: microdontia, incisal attrition
	• Crown lengthening
	  ◦ Diagnosis: altered passive eruption, dentoalveolar extrusion
	• Connective tissue grafting:
	  ◦ Diagnosis: long clinical crown

Fig. 21. Global diagnosis concept.[4–6]

- The 6 treatment options:
  1. Orthognathic surgery:
     - Global Diagnosis: VME
       - Primary treatment: maxillary Le Fort I impaction
       - Alternative treatment: Botox
       - Alternative treatment: crown lengthening and restorative dentistry.
     - Global Diagnosis: VMD: maxillary downfracture, bilateral sagittal split osteotomy (BSSO)
     - Global Diagnosis: angle class II or class III malocclusion
       - Primary Treatment: orthognathic and orthodontics.
  2. Plastic surgery:
     - Global Diagnosis: short upper lip
       - Primary treatment: Botox and lip fillers
       - Secondary treatment: behavior modification.
     - Global Diagnosis: long upper lip
       - Primary treatment: lip lift
     - Global Diagnosis: hypermobile upper lip
       - Primary treatment: Botox
       - Secondary treatment: plastic surgery, behavior modification
     - Global Diagnosis: hypomobile upper lip:
       - Primary treatment: Botox of depressor muscles

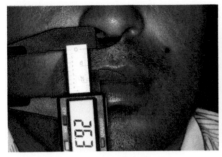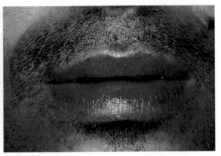

Fig. 22. Long upper lip resulting in no incisal edge display.

3. Orthodontics:
   - Global Diagnosis: dentoalveolar extrusion
     - Primary treatment: orthodontic intrusion, restorative dentistry
   - Global Diagnosis angle class I or class II malocclusion.
     - Primary treatment: orthodontics, orthognathic if needed.
4. Restorations
   - Global Diagnosis: microdontia.
     - Primary treatment: restorative such as veneers, crowns, or composites
   - Global Diagnosis: incisal attrition.
     - Primary treatment: restorative such as veneers, crowns, or composites
5. Crown lengthening:
   - Global Diagnosis: altered passive eruption
     - Primary treatment: esthetic crown lengthening is completed from facial line angle to line angle 3 mm apical to the CEJ.
   - Global Diagnosis: dentoalveolar extrusion
     - Primary treatment: functional crown lengthening is performed to correct the concave gingiva followed by restorative dentistry.
6. Connective tissue grafting:
   - Global Diagnosis: long clinical crown
     - Primary treatment: soft tissue grafting to correct the recession
     - Secondary treatment: restorative dentistry with pink porcelain if needed

It is important to note that alternative treatment plans can be proposed if the patient does not want to proceed with the "ideal" plan, especially in the case of orthognathic surgery. Even though a La-Forte 1 might be indicated, an alternative plan such as crown

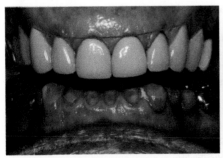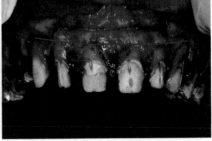

Fig. 23. U-shaped gingiva and bone in dentoalveolar extrusion of maxillary anterior teeth. Treatment is functional crown lengthening.

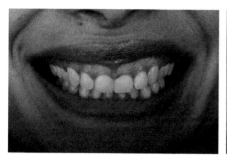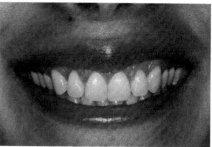

Fig. 24. Altered passive eruption treated with esthetic crown lengthening.

lengthening, Botox, and restorative might be enough to address the patient's esthetic concern; this is the power of digital planning, where the patient can visualize the end result of several plans and mock-ups and go with an informed decision. As with all treatment plans, the pros and cons need to be discussed with the patient. Care should be taken not to compromise the final result when selecting an alternative plan.

SMILE DESIGN TREATMENT PLANNING

Rationale: the 2 treatment planning concepts outlined earlier provide the practitioner with very powerful tools to guide planning advanced interdisciplinary cases. It is the authors' opinion that these 2 concepts can be merged into a more inclusive comprehensive treatment plan philosophy focused on the concepts of *Digital Smile Design* with *Global Diagnosis* and *FGTP*. This proposed concept is termed *Smile Design Treatment Planning (SDTP)* and provides the practitioner with a treatment sequence when dealing with smile design cases. Once the ideal smile is designed, the clinician uses the decision trees discussed later to decide treatment options. Because of the novelty of this concept, changes will be made in the future to address emerging concepts.

Nine steps for SDTP:
1. Data acquisition phase
2. Airway analysis
3. Facial analysis
4. OVD and TMJ analysis
5. Lip analysis
6. Dental analysis
7. Gingival analysis
8. Mandibular arch and occlusal analysis
9. Virtual treatment analysis
- Step 1: data acquisition phase:
  - *Phase summary:* during this phase, the clinician collects diagnostic data for case analysis. These data are used to construct a virtual patient for digital treatment planning. An *SDTP* checklist is also used to provide clinical data (**Fig. 25**).
  - *Requirements:*
    - 5 DSD photos: frontal smile with teeth apart, frontal retracted with teeth apart, profile at rest, profile at smile, and 12 o'clock smile view[54]
    - Repose picture at physiologic rest position (PRP)

- Video of the patient in repose, full smile, spontaneous smile, phonetics
- Kois Dento-Facial Analyzer or digital facebow.
- STLs at current OVD and proposed OVD
- SDTP checklist.

Optional data: facial scan, cone beam computed tomography (for implant planning, guided crown lengthening), cephalometric (orthognathic, orthodontics, and airway analysis), Viewing/Design Software—DSD, Smilefy, Exocad, 3Shape Trios, BlueSky-Bio (Free), MeshMixer (Free)—or other applicable alternatives.

- Step 2: airway analysis
  - *Phase summary:* during this phase, the dentist screens the patient for possible airway involvement. This involves an extraoral and intraoral clinical examination, sleep questionnaire, and possible use of HRPO if airway issues are suspected (discussed earlier). OVD is also assessed at this phase and whether the airway would benefit from increasing the OVD. Airway analysis is also integrated into some of the following steps. Possible airway changes must be considered in each step of SDTP.
- Step 3: facial analysis (**Fig. 26**)
  - *Phase summary:* during this phase, the face is analyzed in repose at PRP in profile and frontal view. Global diagnosis rules are followed.
    - In the frontal view: if the middle:lower face is 1:1 then face proportions are normal. If the lower third is longer then the diagnosis is VME, and the primary treatment is La-Forte 1 impaction. If the middle face is longer then the diagnosis is VMD, and the primary treatment is maxillary downfracture, BSSO.[7]
    - The facial flow is also analyzed in this view and decided whether it is perpendicular or curved.
    - In profile, Rickett's line is used as a reference. If the lower lip is greater than 2 mm posterior, then the face is convex, and the patient is class II. The

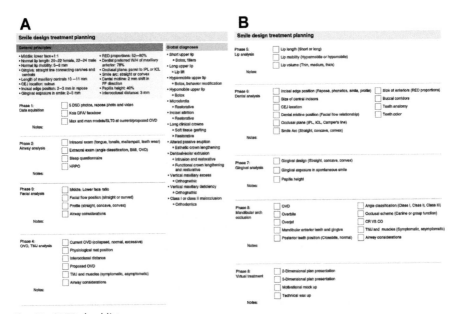

Fig. 25. SDTP checklist.

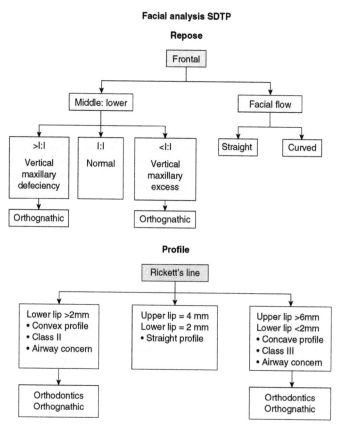

Fig. 26. Facial analysis in SDTP and treatment options.

dentist should be aware of possible airway issues in class II patients due to decreased airway volume.[55] In addition, if the OVD is increased, care should be taken whether to restore the patient in centric relation (CR) or centric occlusion (CO). Restoring a class I or class II patient in CR could worsen airway issues by decreasing airway volume due to the posterior reposition of the mandible. An airway analysis should be conducted with provisional restorations or splint at an open OVD if CR will be used to examine airway volume.[56] If the lower lip is less than 2 mm posterior to the line, then the face is concave (class III), and orthodontics and orthognathic surgery should be considered. Opening the OVD could improve the overbite/overjet relationship for these patients. In some class III patients, the maxilla is deficient and airway volume is decreased.[57]

- *Step 4: OVD and TMJ analysis* (**Fig. 27**)
  - *Phase summary:* once facial and airway analysis is complete, the clinician can now assess the patient's OVD. There are several methods to determine the PRR and OVD.[58] Facial esthetics can be used as a guide to determine the OVD. The accepted interocclusal distance (IOD) is 3 mm but can be a range as noted in a recent study.[59] If the patient has greater IOD, the clinician can use several methods to determine a new OVD such as splint or leaf gauge. The clinician also needs to take into consideration the airway and the patient's

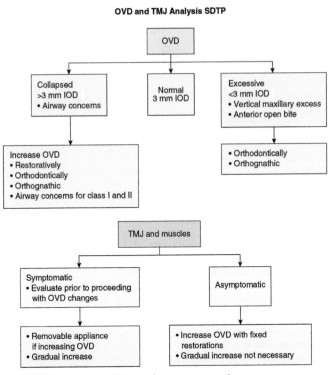

Fig. 27. OVD and TMJ analysis in SDTP and treatment options.

Angle classification as discussed earlier. If the OVD is excessive such as in cases of anterior open bite or VME, then orthognathic surgery and orthodontics are recommended to decrease OVD. TMJ and muscles also need to be assessed during this phase. There is strong clinical evidence that the stomatognathic system can adapt to changes in OVD.[59] However, care should be taken on patients with existing TMD when considering changing the OVD. TMD and muscle issues should be addressed prior. It is also recommended to use a removable appliance to increase the OVD gradually before considering irreversible procedures.[60]

- *Step 5: lip analysis* (**Fig. 28**)
  - *Phase summary:* during this phase, the length, volume, and mobility of the lip are analyzed.
    - Lip length: normal lip length is 20 to 22 for women and 22 to 24 for men. A short lip is to be treated with Botox, whereas a long lip can be treated with a lip lift procedure.
    - Lip mobility: normal mobility is 6 to 8 mm. A hypermobile lip is treated with Botox, whereas a hypomobile lip can be treated with Botox and smile exercises.
    - Lip volume: thin lips are treated with lip fillers.
- Step 6: dental analysis
  - *Phase summary:* during this phase, the position, size, midline, occlusal plane, smile arc, shape, and color are established.

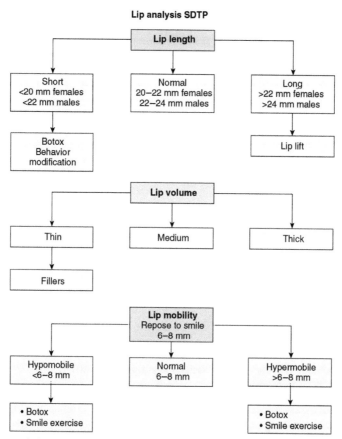

Fig. 28. Lip analysis in SDTP and treatment options.

- Incisal edge position: In a patient with normal lip length and facial proportions the maxillary central incisal edge position is analyzed in repose. In the frontal position, there should be 2 to 3 mm of the incisal display. Phonetics is also used to analyze incisal edge position. The normal position is for the incisal edge to touch the wet-dry border during F sounds. If the incisal display is greater or less, then orthodontics or restorative are considered to correct the position. In the profile view: the nasolabial angle is assessed to evaluate the anterior-posterior position of the maxillary centrals. The normal angle is 90° to 95° in men and 95° to 115° in women. A wider angle or narrower angle can be corrected with orthodontics or restorative (**Fig. 29**).

The following are analyzed in full spontaneous smile with the following assumptions. Any variations need to be taken into consideration.

- Normal lip mobility
- Normal facial proportions
- CEJ is detected in the sulcus. If not, the Global Diagnosis is APE and gingival analysis should be completed first.

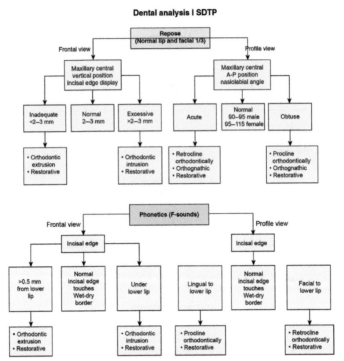

Fig. 29. Incisal edge position analysis, facial analysis phase of SDTP.

○ Size of maxillary centrals: the average size is 10 to 11 mm. Short teeth indicate microdontia or incisal wear and are treated restoratively. Longer teeth with exposed CEJ are treated restoratively or with soft tissue grafting (**Fig. 30**).

○ Dental midline position: once the centrals are set, the dental midline is analyzed in reference to the facial flow. Up to 2 mm deviation is considered esthetic. If the flow is straight, the midline should be parallel. In cases where the flow is curved, the midline angulation should flow in the same direction as the flow toward the green side. Deviations can be treated with orthodontics or restorative (see **Fig. 30**).

○ Occlusal plane: the horizontal plane should be set parallel to the IPL. In cases where the IPL and ICL are not parallel, the ICL is recommended. The transverse plane is set parallel to Camper's line. Variations are treated with orthodontics, orthognathic, or restorative (see **Fig. 30**).

○ Smile arc: straight or convex smile arcs are recommended. If a more dominant smile is desired, the incisal step between the laterals and the centrals is made to be steeper. The smile arc should follow the lower lip. In the case of a concave smile arc, the treatment options are extrusion of the incisors with orthodontics or restorative dentistry to make the teeth longer. The clinician must consider how this would affect OVD, overjet, overbite, incisal edge display in repose, and envelop of function as discussed later (see **Fig. 30**).

○ Size of anterior teeth: once the size of the maxillary centrals is established, the RED proportions and Chu guidelines are used to decide on the size of the remaining anterior teeth. The RED proportions vary between 62% and 80% depending on the gender and size of the patient. If the teeth are wider than

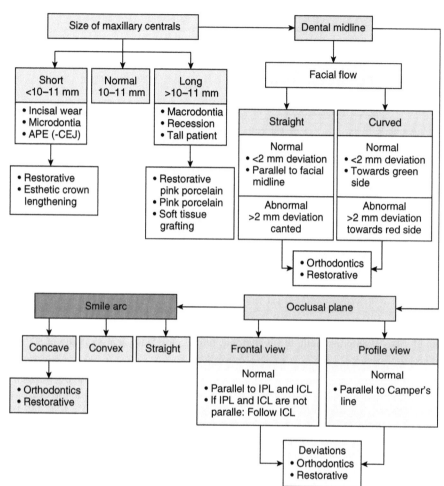

Dental analysis II SDTP

Fig. 30. Size of maxillary centrals, position of dental midline, occlusal plane orientation, smile arc position. Facial analysis phase of SDTP.

desired, orthodontics or restorative options are considered. If the teeth are narrower than desired and diastemas are present, restorative options can be used to close the contacts. If diastemas are absent, that means that the maxillary arch is narrow, and the buccal corridors are wide. Decrease in airway volume is a concern in these situations, and palatal expansion is recommended (**Fig. 31**).

○ Tooth anatomy: the anatomy of teeth is then decided with variables such as line angles, contact length, height of contour, embrasures, texture, and shape. A natural or artificial library can be used (see **Fig. 31**).

○ Tooth color: the color of the teeth is altered either by bleaching protocols or by restorative options. In cases of dark teeth that will be restored with translucent ceramics, the stump shade needs to be identified (see **Fig. 31**).

• *Step 7: gingival analysis* (**Fig. 32**)

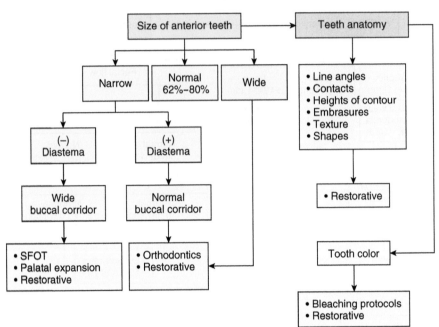

Dental analysis II SDTP

Fig. 31. Size of anterior teeth, tooth anatomy, tooth color, facial analysis phase of SDTP.

- *Phase summary:* once the teeth are set, the gingival architecture is analyzed. If the gingiva is convex when connecting the maxillary anteriors and the maxillary centrals are in the correct position, there is either recession of the maxillary incisors that needs to be treated with soft tissue grafting or APE that can be treated with esthetic crown lengthening. If the gingiva is concave, the diagnosis is DAE, and the treatment options are orthodontic intrusion or functional crown lengthening and restorative. Gingival exposure in full smile should be *2 to 3 mm.* Excessive gingival exposure can be due to hypermobile lip, short lip, VME, or APE if CEJ is not detectable. If gingival exposure is deficient, reasons could be long lip, hypomobile lip, VMD, or recession. Treatment options for these have been described earlier. Papillary height ideally is 40%. If it is more than 40%, crown lengthening and changing the shape of the teeth can be done if desired. If papilla height is less than 40% and black triangles are present: longer contacts are recommended. If black triangles are absent, then changing the shape of the teeth and soft tissue grafting may lead to an increase in height of the papilla.
- *Step 8: mandibular arch and occlusion analysis*
  - *Phase summary:* once the maxillary arch is set, the mandibular arch and occlusion are established.
    - Mandibular incisal edge is decided at the proposed vertical from step 4. If the overbite is excessive, then the OVD needs to be increased or orthodontics or orthognathic surgery is considered. If the overbite is reduced, the clinician should consider reducing the proposed OVD if possible while considering the airway. If restorative space is needed, then orthodontics or orthognathic surgery should be considered. For class I and class II patients, increasing the

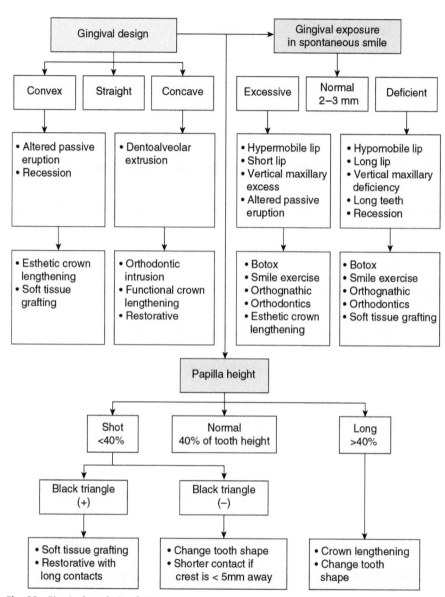

Fig. 32. Gingival analysis of SDTP.

OVD will increase the overjet, resulting in bulkier lingual restorations of the maxillary anteriors or longer restorations on the mandibular anteriors to obtain coupling.[58] Longer mandibular anterior crowns can affect the envelope of function, anterior guidance, and esthetics. Steeper interincisal angles should be avoided to prevent functional and structural damage.[58] *As a general rule, increasing the OVD by 1 mm in the posterior decreases the overbite by 2 mm, and the overjet increases by 1.3 mm*[58] (**Fig. 33**).

Mandibular arch and occlusion analysis SDTP

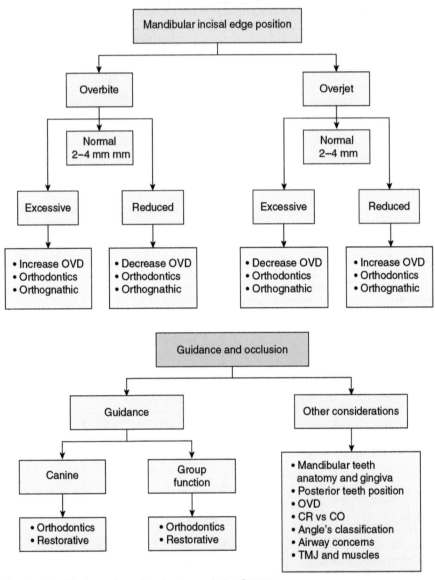

Fig. 33. Mandibular arch and occlusion analysis of SDTP.

■ Guidance and occlusion: the guidance is then established to achieve anterior and canine guidance if possible. The mandibular posterior teeth are set in occlusion with the maxillary posterior at the correct OVD and Angle classification with mutually protected occlusion and no posterior interferences. In cases where canine guidance is not possible, group function can be considered to share the load.[61]

■ Teeth shape and gingiva: the shape and size of the mandibular teeth are related to the maxillary teeth using Chu's guidelines. Moreover, the gingival architecture follows the same guidelines outlined earlier for the maxillary gingiva in terms of design. DAE is common in patients with sleep apnea or

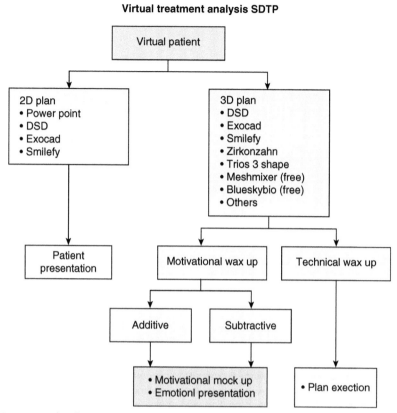

Virtual treatment analysis SDTP

Fig. 34. Dentoalveolar extrusion of the mandibular anteriors. Patient treated with functional crown lengthening of lower anteriors and crowns.

patients with mandibular wear (**Fig. 34**). The treatment of choice is functional crown lengthening and restorative or orthodontic intrusion and restorative.
- *Step 9: virtual treatment phase* (**Fig. 35**)
  ○ *Phase summary:* once the virtual plan is established, the patient is presented with 2 plans. The 2-dimensional plan is based on a photographic mock-up using traditional applications such as PowerPoint or contemporary digital technology such as DSD, SmileFy, or Exocad. During this phase, the clinician involves the patient in step-by-step plan such as selection of teeth library, shape, sizes incisal edge display, gingival design, and other variables. The more powerful part of the virtual treatment is based on the 3-dimensional design with the diagnostic wax-up. Two types of wax-ups should be created: a motivational wax-up and a technical wax-up. The motivational wax-up is used to simulate the final result in the patient's mouth. This is an additive wax-up and can be used as a diagnostic tool by the dentist to evaluate occlusal plane, OVD, gingival display, and other variables. If the mock-up is subtractive, then a computer-simulated plan will have to be used instead. The technical wax-up is used when the actual treatment starts; this is not additive and is more anatomic. This step is explained in more detail when discussing DSD.[62]

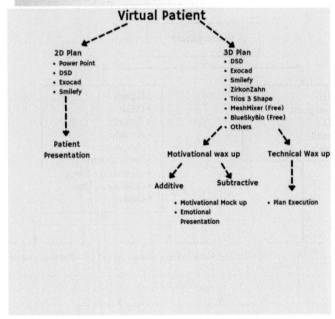

Fig. 35. Virtual treatment phase of SDTP.

SUMMARY

Smile design is an interdisciplinary process that requires a detailed understanding of the principles outlined earlier. A thorough understanding of treatment planning principles and options is essential when dealing with smile design cases. Digital technology has allowed us to improve our interdisciplinary capabilities and deliver a more predictable outcome with better quality control. In this book, each article discusses the specifics of different diagnoses and treatment options outlined in this article. The overall goal is to provide the smile designers with a comprehensive overview of treatment options when constructing a new smile.

CLINICS CARE POINTS

- Smile Design is multi-factorial and depends on a thorough understanding of all components of the smile: Face, gingiva, lips and teeth.

REFERENCES

1. Darwin C. In: Murray J, Street A, editors. The expression of the emotions in man and animals. 1872. Available at: https://pure.mpg.de/rest/items/item_2309885/component/file_2309884/content. Accessed February 8, 2022.
2. Harker L, Keltner D. Expressions of positive emotion in women's college yearbook pictures and their relationship to personality and life outcomes across adulthood. J Pers Soc Psychol 2001;80(1):112–24.
3. Beall AE. Can a new smile make you look more intelligent and successful? Dent Clin North Am 2007;51(2):289–97.

4. Davis NC. Smile Design. Dent Clin N Am 2007;51(2):299–318.

5. Machado AW. 10 commandments of smile esthetics. Dent Press J Orthod 2014; 19(4):136–57.

6. Mahn E, Sampaio CS, Silva BP da, et al. Comparing the use of static versus dynamic images to evaluate a smile. J Prosthet Dent 2020;123(5):739–46.

7. Robbins JW, Rouse JS. Global diagnosis A new vision of dental diagnosis and treatment planning, 4. Quintessence; 2016. https://doi.org/10.25241/stomaeduj. 2017.4(3).bookreview.2.

8. Meiyappan N, Tamizharasi S, Senthilkumar KP, et al. Natural head position: An overview. J Pharm Bioallied Sci 2015;7(Suppl 2):S424–7.

9. Fradeani M. Esthetic rehabilitation in fixed prosthodontics, 1. Quintessence Publishing Co Inc; 2004. Available at: http://www.quintpub.com/display_detail.php3? psku=BI004#. Accessed February 13, 2022.

10. Arroyo-Cruz G, Orozco-Varo A, Vilches-Ahumada M, et al. Comparative analysis of smile aesthetics between top celebrity smile and a Southern European population. J Prosthet Dent 2021. https://doi.org/10.1016/j.prosdent.2021.03.019.

11. Silva BP, Jiménez-Castellanos E, Finkel S, et al. Layperson's preference regarding orientation of the transverse occlusal plane and commissure line from the frontal perspective. J Prosthet Dent 2017;117(4):513–6.

12. Silva BP, Mahn E, Stanley K, et al. The facial flow concept: an organic orofacial analysis—the vertical component. J Prosthet Dent 2018;121(2):189–94.

13. The glossary of prosthodontic terms ninth edition. J Prosthet Dent 2017;117(5): e1–105.

14. Priest G, Wilson MG. An evaluation of benchmarks for esthetic orientation of the occlusal plane. J Prosthodont 2017;26(3):216–23.

15. Mazurkiewicz P, Oblizajek M, Rzeszowska J, et al. Determining the occlusal plane: a literature review. Cranio 2019;1–7. https://doi.org/10.1080/08869634. 2019.1703093.

16. Levine JB, Finkel S. Smile design integrating esthetics and function. vol. 2. Levine JB, editor. ELSEVIER; 2016;1:1–42.

17. Farias F de O, Ennes JP, Zorzatto JR. Aesthetic value of the relationship between the shapes of the face and permanent upper central incisor. Int J Dent 2010; 2010:561957.

18. Gurel G, Paolucci B, Lliev G, et al. The art and creation of a personalized smile: visual identity of the smile. Quintessence: VIS; 2019.

19. Sforza C, Laino A, D'Alessio R, et al. Soft-tissue facial characteristics of attractive italian women as compared to normal women. Angle Orthod 2009;79(1):17–23.

20. Stanley K, Caligiuri M, Schlichting LH, et al. Lip lifting: unveiling dental beauty. Int J Esthetic Dent 2017;12(1):108–14.

21. Fink B, Neave N, Seydel H. Male facial appearance signals physical strength to women. Am J Hum Biol 2007;19(1):82–7.

22. Roe P, Rungcharassaeng K, Kan JYK, et al. The influence of upper lip length and lip mobility on maxillary incisal exposure. Am J Esthetic Dentistry 2012.

23. Tosun H, Kaya B. Effect of maxillary incisors, lower lip, and gingival display relationship on smile attractiveness. Am J Orthod Dentofac 2020;157(3):340–7.

24. Sarver DM, Ackerman MB. Dynamic smile visualization and quantification: part 2. smile analysis and treatment strategies. Am J Orthod Dentofac 2003;124(2): 116–27.

25. Wang C, Hu W, Liang L, et al. Esthetics and smile-related characteristics assessed by laypersons. J Esthet Restor Dent 2018;30(2):136–45.

26. Crawford RWI, Tredwin C, Moles D, et al. Smile esthetics: the influence of posterior maxillary gingival margin position. J Prosthodont 2012;21(4):270–8.
27. Chu SJ, Tan JH, Stappert CFJ, et al. Gingival zenith positions and levels of the maxillary anterior dentition. J Esthet Restor Dent 2009;21(2):113–20.
28. Hochman MN, Chu SJ, Tarnow DP. Maxillary anterior papilla display during smiling: a clinical study of the interdental smile line. Int J Periodontics Restorative Dent 2012;32(4):375–83.
29. Salama H, Salama MA, Garber D, et al. The interproximal height of bone: a guidepost to predictable aesthetic strategies and soft tissue contours in anterior tooth replacement. Pract Periodontics Aesthet Dent 1998;. https://pubmed.ncbi.nlm.nih.gov/10093558/.
30. Al-Habahbeh R, Al-Shammout R, Al-Jabrah O, et al. The effect of gender on tooth and gingival display in the anterior region at rest and during smiling. Eur J Esthetic Dent 2009;4(4):382–95.
31. Gaikwad S. Influence of smile arc and buccal corridors on facial attractiveness: a cross-sectional study. J Clin Diagn Res 2016. https://doi.org/10.7860/jcdr/2016/19013.8436.
32. Pound E. Utilizing speech to simplify a personalized denture service. J Prosthet Dent 1970;24(6):586–600.
33. Proffit WR. Fields H.W.Sarver D.M.Contemporary orthodontics. 6th ed. Philadelphia, PA: Elsevier; 2018. p. 156–75.
34. Al-Johany SS, Alqahtani AS, Alqahtani FY, et al. Evaluation of different esthetic smile criteria - PubMed. Int J Prosthodont 2011;. https://pubmed.ncbi.nlm.nih.gov/21210007/.
35. Wolfart S, Thormann H, Freitag S, et al. Assessment of dental appearance following changes in incisor proportions. Eur J Oral Sci 2005;113(2):159–65.
36. German DS, Chu SJ, Furlong ML, et al. Simplifying optimal tooth-size calculations and communications between practitioners. Am J Orthod Dentofac 2016;150(6):1051–5.
37. Correa BD, Bittencourt MAV, Machado AW. Influence of maxillary canine gingival margin asymmetries on the perception of smile esthetics among orthodontists and laypersons. Am J Orthod Dentofac 2014;145(1):55–63.
38. Levin EI. Dental esthetics and the golden proportion. J Prosthet Dent 1978;40(3):244–52.
39. Mahshid M, Khoshvaghti A, Varshosaz M, et al. Evaluation of "Golden Proportion" in individuals with an esthetic smile. J Esthet Restor Dent 2004;16(3):185–92.
40. Ward DH. Proportional smile design. Dent Clin N Am 2015;59(3):623–38.
41. Reis PMP, Lima P, Garcia FCP, et al. Effect of maxillary median diastema on the esthetics of a smile. Am J Orthod Dentofac 2020;158(4):e37–42.
42. Prasad KN, Sabrish S, Mathew S, et al. Comparison of the influence of dental and facial aesthetics in determining overall attractiveness. Int Orthod 2018;16(4):684–97.
43. Cruz GA, Varo AO, Luna FM, et al. Esthetic assessment of celebrity smiles. J Prosthet Dent 2021;125(1):146–50.
44. Kokich VO, Kokich VG, Kiyak HA. Perceptions of dental professionals and laypersons to altered dental esthetics: asymmetric and symmetric situations. Am J Orthod Dentofac 2006;130(2):141–51.
45. Ferreira JB, Silva LE da, Caetano MT de O, et al. Perception of midline deviations in smile esthetics by laypersons. Dent Press J Orthod 2016;21(06):51–7.
46. Murro BD, Gallusi G, Nardi R, et al. The relationship of tooth shade and skin tone and its influence on the smile attractiveness. J Esthet Restor Dent 2020;32(1):57–63.

47. Kumar MV, Ahila SC, Devi SS. The science of anterior teeth selection for a completely edentulous patient: a literature review. J Indian Prosthodont Soc 2011;11(1):7–13.
48. Roblee RD. Interdisciplinary dentofacial therapy (IDT): a comprehensive approach to optimal patient care. Quintessence: Quintessence Publishing Co Inc; 1994.
49. Blatz MB, Chiche G, Bahat O, et al. Evolution of aesthetic dentistry. J Dent Res 2019;98(12):1294–304.
50. Spear FM, Kokich, Mathews VG. Interdisciplinary management of anterior dental estheticsSpear. JADA 2006.
51. Sabbah A. An introduction to contemporary treatment planning.pdf. Metlife, ed. 2021. Available at: https://metdental.ecepartners.com/coursereview.aspx? url=1902%2FHTML%2FAn_Introduction_to_Contemporary_Treatment_Planning %2Findex.html&scid=15011. Accessed February 20, 2022.
52. Rouse J. Airway and 3D treatment planning - spear education. 2019. https://www. speareducation.com/spear-review/2019/11/airway-and-3d-treatment-planning. Accessed February 10, 2022.
53. Masoud AI, Jackson GW, Carley DW. Sleep and airway assessment: a review for dentists. Cranio 2016;35(4):206–22.
54. Yoshinga C. Yoshinga. DSD photo and video protocol. Available at: https://www. dsdplanningcenter.com/pdf/dsd-video-photo-protocol.pdf. Accessed February 20, 2022.
55. Kirjavainen M, Kirjavainen T. Upper airway dimensions in class II malocclusion. Angle Orthod 2007;77(6):1046–53.
56. Harrell WE, Tatum T, Koslin M. Is centric relation always the position of choice for TMDs? case report of how TMD and airway dimension may be associated. Compendium 2017. Available at: https://www.aegisdentalnetwork.com/cced/2017/04/ is-centric-relation-always-the-position-of-choice-for-tmds-case-report-of-how-tmd-and-airway-dimension-may-be-associated. Accessed February 20, 2022.
57. Chen X, Liu D, Liu J, et al. Three-dimensional evaluation of the upper airway morphological changes in growing patients with skeletal class III malocclusion treated by protraction headgear and rapid palatal expansion: a comparative research. PLoS One 2015;10(8):e0135273.
58. Calamita M, Coachman C, Sesma N, et al. Occlusal vertical dimension: treatment planning decisions and management considerations. Int J Esthetic Dent 2019; 14(2):166–81.
59. Goldstein G, Goodacre C, MacGregor K. Occlusal vertical dimension: best evidence consensus statement. J Prosthodont 2021;30(S1):12–9.
60. Abduo J, Lyons K. Clinical considerations for increasing occlusal vertical dimension: a review. Aust Dent J 2012;57(1):2–10.
61. Miralles R. Canine-guide occlusion and group function occlusion are equally acceptable when restoring the dentition. J Évid Based Dent Pract 2016; 16(1):41–3.
62. Coachman C, Georg R, Bohner L, et al. Chairside 3D digital design and trial restoration workflow. J Prosthet Dent 2020;124(5):514–20.

An Overview of Maxillofacial Approaches to Smile Design

Pooyan Sadr-Eshkevari, DDS, MD*, Robert L. Flint, DMD, MD,
Brian Alpert, DDS, FICD

KEYWORDS

- Oral and maxillofacial surgery • Facial anatomy • Smile • Orthognathic surgery
- Cosmetic surgery • Facial cosmetics • Smile design • Surgical anatomy

KEY POINTS

- In an ideal smile, the entire maxillary premolar to premolar is visible, lower lip slightly touches the maxillary incisal edges, and the lip curvatures is parallel to that of the maxillary incisal edges.
- For an average-sized face, the philtrum should ideally be 10 to 11 mm wide and 12 to 15 mm in length.
- Zygomaticus major is the main determinant of smile dynamics and the basis for the Rubin classification of Mona Lisa, cupid, and complex smiles.
- Gummy smile may be caused by vertical maxillary excess, anterior dentoalveolar extrusion, altered passive eruption, gingival hypertrophy, short upper lip, hypermobile upper lip, asymmetric upper lip, or a combination of these. The differentiation of the cause is crucial in proper management.
- Chemical (neuromodulator like Botox) or physical lysis of Depressor Alae Nasi may correct hyperactive and/or upper lip both of which may correct gummy smile.

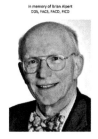

In memory of Brian Alpert
DDS, FACS, FACD, FICD

It was only a sunny smile, and little it cost in the giving, but like morning light it scattered the night and made the day worth living.

— F. Scott Fitzgerald

Oral and Maxillofacial Surgery Department, University of Louisville, Louisville, KY, USA
* Corresponding author. Oral and Maxillofacial Surgery Department, University of Louisville School of Dentistry, 501 South Preston Street, Room 148L, Louisville, KY 40292.
E-mail address: Pseshk01@louisville.edu

Dent Clin N Am 66 (2022) 343–360
https://doi.org/10.1016/j.cden.2022.02.001
0011-8532/22/© 2022 Elsevier Inc. All rights reserved.

INTRODUCTION

A perfect smile is an esthetic harmony of mild imperfections. It is the result of a fluid interplay of volumes, angles, and dimensions. The static bony and dental structures and the dynamic soft tissue components of the middle and the lower facial thirds dictate the symmetry and the beauty of the smile.[1] Aside from the occlusal, dental, and gingival components, the main factors influencing the smile are the lip line and volume, the smile arch and symmetry, the upper lip curvature, the lateral negative space, and the skeletal relationship of the maxilla and mandible relative to each other and the skull.[1]

In an ideal smile, the entire maxillary premolar to premolar extension should show. Also, the lower lip should slightly touch the anterior maxillary incisal edges and the lip curvatures should be parallel to that of the maxillary incisal edges. Deviation from these ideals may affect the beauty of smile. Clinically significant smile asymmetry may involve the perioral and labial "frame," the dentogingival "display," and/or their relative positioning. For instance, a gummy smile is a great example of smile disharmony with several possible causes. These include malocclusions, short tooth syndrome, skeletal deformities, and neuromuscular deficiencies. Aside from the static measurements, recent research has suggested that smile asymmetry, if present, is minimal at rest but increases exponentially over the duration of the smile. This fluctuating asymmetry exists within and between individuals adding to the complexity of smile design. Clinical rather than mathematical (Procrustes) midline seems to be more appropriate for the analysis of this fluctuation, especially in individuals with clinically significant asymmetry at rest.[2]

Although the restorative dentist, the periodontist, and the orthodontist have made tremendous breakthroughs in the betterment of the dental, gingival, and occlusal components of the smile, the oral and maxillofacial surgeon (OMS) has been privileged with the skills to alter the musculoskeletal, neural, and cutaneous structures drastically and efficiently to improve facial animation and esthetics. Evidence shows that the OMS has the same "eye" for the small smile asymmetries as the orthodontist.[3] An interdisciplinary approach to smile management would then be the most desirable especially when dealing with the more complex anomalies. This article provides an overview of the scope of OMS in smile design and helps understand the need for referral to OMS when indicated.

GROSS ANATOMY

The anatomy of the upper and lower lips and their associated structures play a crucial role in smile esthetics. Upper lip starts from the base of the nose superiorly and the two nasolabial folds laterally and extends inferiorly to the lower border of the vermillion. The two paramedian elevations in the upper vermillion, known as the Cupid's bow, follow the philtral columns. The philtral dimple sits between these columns. The lower lip extends from the superior edge of the lower vermillion to the oral commissures laterally and the inverted U-shaped labiomental crease inferiorly. For an average-sized face, the philtrum should ideally be 10 to 11 mm wide and 12 to 15 mm in length. Aging is associated with thinning of the vermilions and elongation of the philtrum.[4]

Another crucial factor in smile esthetics is the nasolabial angle (NLA). NLA is defined as the angle between the columella and a line intersecting the subnasale and the most anterior point of the upper lip, known as labrale superius. The protrusion of the lips and the outlines of nasal tip are the main determinants of NLA esthetics.[5] According to Brown and Guyuron,[6] NLA in the eye of the cosmetic surgeon is ideally 93.9 to 97.3

for males and 96.8 to 100.2 for females. According to Armijo and colleagues[7] these values are consistent with 93.4 to 98.5 and 95.5 to 100.1 in males and females, respectively, as judged by the general public.

SURGICAL ANATOMY

The dental and occlusal determinants of smile are discussed in depth elsewhere in this issue. Here we focus on the other pertinent components, namely the musculocutane-ous and the skeletal anatomy. These intricacies become important in cosmetic and orthognathic surgeries, facial rejuvenation using neurotoxins, and facial reanimation in paralysis cases. An in-depth discussion of the surgical anatomy is outside the scope of this article. Rather, we highlight the most pertinent anatomic considerations.

The main determinants of the dynamics of the smile are three groups of muscles categorized based on their insertion. Group one, which is the most important group, inserts into modiolus and includes orbicularis oris (OO), buccinators, levator anguli oris (LAO), and depressor anguli oris, zygomaticus major (ZM), and risorius (**Fig. 1**).[8] ZM is the major determinant of smile dynamics with four major anatomic variations based on cadaver studies of Shim and colleagues (**Fig. 2**).[9] In type I, which is seen in more than half of the cases, the superficial muscle bands blend with the LAO, whereas the deep muscle bands blend into the buccinator. Cadaver studies by Elvan and colleagues[10] have shown ZM to be mostly bandlike (51%), and less commonly fanlike (34%) or bifid (13%). They also reported that the position of ZM relative to the OO is variable. OO either overlaps (52%) or sides (48%) ZM.

Rubin[11] was the first to come up with a smile classification in 1974. He categorized smile patterns based on the function of ZM. A commissure smile (also known as Mona Lisa smile) in his classification describes a more pronounced upward traction of the commissures compared with the Cupid's bow. A cuspid smile (also known as canine

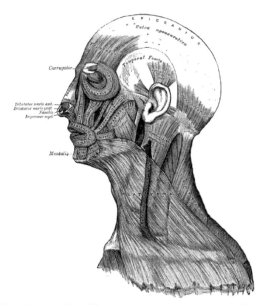

Fig. 1. Muscles of facial expression. (*from* Gray's Anatomy, plate 378)

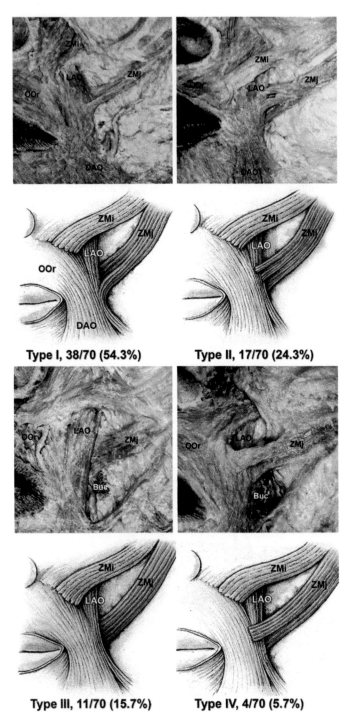

Fig. 2. Four anatomic patterns of the zygomaticus major muscle. (*Top left*) Type I: the superficial muscle band is blended with the LAO, whereas deep muscle band blends into the buccinator and LAO, deep to LAO. (*Top right*) Type II: the superficial band is blended into

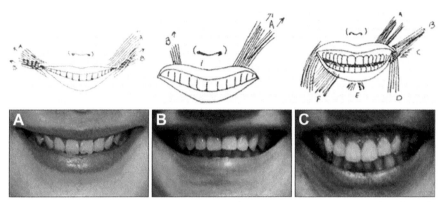

Fig. 3. Rubin smile classification. (*A*) The corner of the mouth, or Mona Lisa smile, where the action of zygomaticus major is dominant. (*B*) The canine smile with the dominance of levator labii superioris. (*C*) The "full denture" smile where no muscle is dominant but all are active and expose the entire dentition. (Top figure reprinted with permission *from* Rubin LR. The anatomy of a smile: its importance in the treatment of facial paralysis. Plast Reconstr Surg. 1974 Apr;53(4):384-7; bottom figure reprinted with permission *from* Liang LZ et al, Analysis of dynamic smile and upper lip curvature in young Chinese. Int J Oral Sci. 2013 Mar;5(1):49-53)

smile) refers to the uniform elevation of the upper lip without an upward movement of the commissures. In the full-denture smile (also known as complex smile) is seen a combination of cuspid smile superiorly and an inferior movement of the lower lip (**Fig. 3**).[12]

ZM is also responsible for the expression of dimples with smile. Dimples may be unilateral or bilateral and are seen in both genders. They are universally known to enhance smile cosmesis. Anatomically, they are caused by bifid ZM, whose fascial strands insert into the dermis and tether the skin while smiling.[13] LAO helps elevate the commissure and refines and augments the effect of ZM. Although ZM pulls the commissure posteriorly, superiorly, and laterally, LAO alters the vector to a more superior direction.[14] The upper lip elevation is caused by the contraction of levator labii superioris (LLS) and the zygomaticus minor.

Another important muscle in smile esthetics and harmony is the depressor septi nasi muscle (DSN), which is further discussed next in the gummy smile section. For more thorough dissection of the surgical anatomy, the authors recommend the anatomy textbooks and the abundant cadaver studies in the maxillofacial literature.

---

the superficial layer of the orbicularis oris (OOr) and the depressor anguli oris (DAO), passing over LAO; the middle band is interlaced into LAO; and the deep band is blended with the buccinator and LAO, deep to LAO. (*Bottom left*) Type III: only a single muscle band passes deep into LAO and also interlaces with the buccinator. (*Bottom right*) Type IV: the superficial muscle band is blended with the OOr and the depressor anguli oris, passing over the LAO and the deep muscle band interlace with buccinator and LAO, deep to LAO. ZMi, zygomaticus minor. (Reprinted with permission *from* Shim KS, et al. An anatomical study of the insertion of the zygomaticus major muscle in humans focused on the muscle arrangement at the corner of the mouth. Plast Reconstr Surg. 2008 Feb;121(2):466-473).

GUMMY SMILE

The most common smile asymmetry is gummy smile, also known as high smile. A gingival show of more than 3 to 4 mm is considered excessive and unesthetic. In an average-sized face, the average length of the upper lip in repose, from subnasale to the upper stomion, is 18 to 23 mm, with males showing higher measurements. When the upper lip is elevated, its length decreases by 20%. This should ideally result in a gingival display of 1 to 2 mm in full smile for females and less for males.[15] High smile may have several causes including vertical maxillary excess (VME), anterior dentoalveolar extrusion, altered passive eruption, gingival hypertrophy, short upper lip, hypermobile upper lip, asymmetric upper lip, or a combination of these.[16,17] Upper lip hypermobility is often caused by the altered anatomy or function of the DSN muscle. The overactivity of this muscle sharpens the NLA in correlation to the activity of LLS alaeque nasi (LLSAN) and OO muscles (**Fig. 4**). Ebrahimi and colleagues[18] in a cadaver study found that unlike the uniform insertion and course of the DSN, its origin may be variable. It is either the periosteum of the maxilla, OO muscle, or floating. Sinno and colleagues[19] in a systematic review of 13 articles, including 175 cadaver specimens and 821 surgically treated patients, determined the most common origin of DSN to be the maxilla and/or OO muscle, and the insertion of the muscle to be the medial crura and adjacent soft tissue.

VME may cause gummy smile despite normal length and mobility of the upper lip. However, a hypoplastic maxillary bone may decrease the ideal tooth display and result in an older-age smile pattern. Also, constriction of the maxilla is likely to result in significant buccal corridor show that is not esthetic. Orthognathic surgery is therefore an important tool in correction of facial and smile esthetics. Of note, upper lip in some individuals unilaterally cants with smiling, which needs to be considered in orthognathic and cosmetic surgeries.[20] Alternatively, camouflage orthodontic procedures may temporarily or permanently help attenuate the discrepancies.[21]

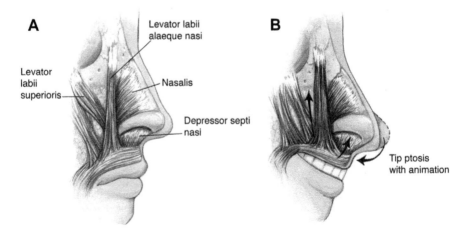

Fig. 4. Overactivity of the depressor septi nasi shortens the upper lip and results in nasal tip ptosis during smile. (*A*) repose. (*B*) smile (Reprinted with permission *from* Ducic, Yadranko, and Robert DeFatta. "Closed rhinoplasty." Operative Techniques in Otolaryngology-Head and Neck Surgery 18.3 (2007): 233-242).

GINGIVOPLASTY

Gingival hypertrophy, lip hyperfunctioning, and maxillary excess are among the most common causes of high smile. Proper diagnosis is therefore crucial because the management requires a well-coordinated collaboration among the restorative dentist, the orthodontist, and the OMS.

An esthetic gingival margin is scalloped, knife-edged, tightly adapted to the tooth surface, and symmetric. The maxillary gingival line ideally follows the upper lip line. Although the gingival margin of central incisors and canines should be at the same level, the lateral incisors should show a more coronally positioned gingival margin.[17] The most apical point of the buccal gingival margin is known as gingival zenith. For mesial incisors, this point ideally is 1 mm distal to the axial inclination. This value ideally is 0.5 mm for lateral incisors and 0 for maxillary canines (coinciding with vertical axis).[22]

Both gingival excess and recession compromise the smile. Gingival hypertrophy, edema, and erythema may cause or worsen high smile.[23] Control of local and systemic factors influencing the gingiva is therefore essential to the success of esthetic smile design. A range of different interventions is available and adequately described elsewhere in this issue and in the literature. Crown-lengthening, orthodontic intrusion, and additive and resective gingival surgeries are the most important gingivoplasty measures.[23] They are done as stand-alone corrective procedures or as an addition to orthognathic surgeries, rhinoplasties, and other cosmetic procedures.

The position of the papillae is also a determinant of smile esthetics, and "black triangles" are considered unfavorable. For OMS, it is generally believed that establishing an adequate distance of 5 mm or less, as described by Tarnow and colleagues,[24] between the interproximal bone crest and the contact point results in adequate papillae formation. A recent systematic review by Roccuzzo and colleagues,[25] however, indicated that this notion is not supported by sufficient evidence. They proposed that

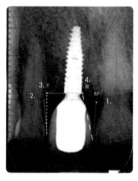

- Interproximal contact point (CP)
- Bone level at the adjacent tooth (BL)
- Inter proximal bone peak (BP)
- Bone level at the reference point at implant level (R)
- Bone level at the implant (Bl)

1. Contact Point - Bone Peak
(Degidi et al 2008; Perez et al 2012; Cosyn et al 2012; Malchiodi et al. 2013)

2. Contact Point - Bone level at the adjacent tooth
(Choquet et al. 2001; Henriksson & Jemt 2004; Palmer et al. 2007; Nisapakultorn et al. 2010; Lops et al 2011; Lops et al 2013; Borges et al. 2014)

3. Contact Point - Reference point (Chang & Wennstrom et al 2013)

4. Contact Point - Bone level at the implant (Henriksson & Jemt 2004; Palmer et al. 2007; Nisapakultorn et al. 2010)

Fig. 5. The selected reference points and the measured distances in the 12 selected studies of the systematic review published by Roccuzzo and colleagues. The vertical distance from the base of the interproximal contact point to the crestal bone level did not seem to affect the interproximal papilla height. Prevention of *black triangle* in implant placement in esthetic zone was more likely to be correlated with the integrity of the periodontal ligament of the tooth. The authors recommended interproximal probing on the adjacent teeth before implant placement to reduce the risk of aesthetic failures. (Reproduced with permission *from* Roccuzzo M, et al. Papilla height in relation to the distance between bone crest and interproximal contact point at single-tooth implants: A systematic review. Clin Oral Implants Res. 2018 Mar;29 Suppl 15:50-61).

adequate embrasure fill between an implant restoration and the adjacent tooth rather depends on the integrity of the periodontal ligament. They recommended interproximal probing on the adjacent teeth before implant placement to reduce the risk of esthetic failure. In another systematic review, they assessed the mucosal fill between the two adjacent implants in anterior maxilla and were unable to define an optimal horizontal distance between two adjacent implants.[26] Around the same time and consistent with their results, the Second Consensus Meeting of the Osteology Foundation concluded that the implant-tooth papilla height mainly depends on the clinical attachment level of the tooth. They were not able to define an optimal horizontal distance between two adjacent implants restored with fixed prostheses to reliably gain adequate papillae height.[27] However, they suggested that lateral bone augmentation is likely to stabilize peri-implant tissue for up to 3 years (**Fig. 5**).[28]

LIP LIFT

OMS often alter the upper lip components to optimize the smile. These modifications are indicated in correcting the maxillary tooth show, everting the upper lip outward and upward to establish a more youthful smile, and augmenting the outlines of the upper lip.[29] Ideal lip augmentation techniques should not only achieve the desired esthetic results but should also provide adequate longevity, low complication rate, and no functional compromise.[30] Moragas and colleagues[31] published a comprehensive systematic review in 2014 summarizing all the nonfilling lip augmentation procedures and assessed their effects. They concluded that indirect lip lift, involving modification of the nasolabial fold tissues, seems to be the preferred method over direct lip lift, which involves excising around the vermilion. Indirect lip lift encompasses a diverse range of techniques including the bullhorn incision, upper lip suspension, double-duck suspension, or the Italian incision, among others. These modalities may have different outcomes and complications. **Fig. 6** presents an illustrated summary of these techniques.

The most widely used indirect lip lift procedure is subnasal lift, or bullhorn lip lift, which shortens the elongated lip and everts the vermillion border. The surgery involves excision of an ellipse of skin and subcutaneous tissue immediately below the base of nostrils. This technique may be done symmetrically or asymmetrically depending on the baseline esthetics, and may complement other cosmetic procedures.[32] The best outcomes are achieved when the ratio of the nasal base width to the upper lip width, from base of nose to the vermillion border, is around 1:2. A smaller ratio may result in undercorrection of the lateral lip lines and is unesthetic. Waldman[33] has explained the procedure in detail and presented some cases in a previous issue, which we recommend for further reference. This procedure has also gained popularity as a gender-confirming surgery, especially for facial feminization. The goals are to reduce the upper lip skin show, to enhance visibility of red vermilion, and to augment pout with minimal scarring.

Several modifications of the upper lip lift are discussed in the literature.[30] Echo and colleagues[34] have described the upper lip suspension technique. This method involves an intranasal incision and using suspension sutures to anchor the upper lip to the anterior nasal spine. Although technically more complex, this technique has the obvious advantage of leaving no trace. The other advantage of this technique is easy reversibility by simply removing the suture intranasally if the patient is not satisfied with the outcomes. Originally explained by Cardim and colleagues,[35] double-duck nasolabial lifting is another method, which combines upper lip and nasal tip rejuvenation. The other advantages are concealed scars and the use of suspension screws to prevent alar ptosis or early relapse.[36] V-Y lip augmentation and its several

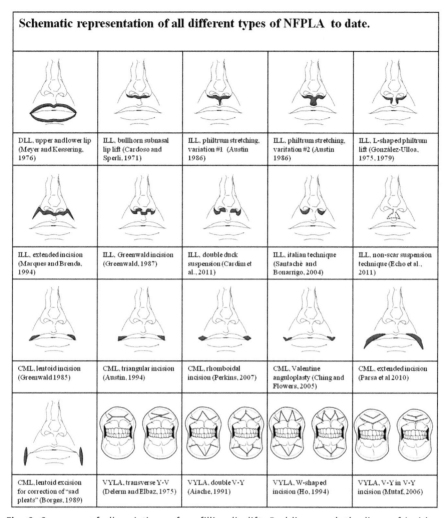

Schematic representation of all different types of NFPLA to date.

DLL, upper and lower lip (Meyer and Kessering, 1976)	ILL, bullhorn subnasal lip lift (Cardoso and Sperli, 1971)	ILL, philtrum stretching, variation #1 (Austin 1986)	ILL, philtrum stretching, varitation #2 (Austin 1986)	ILL, L-shaped philtrum lift (González-Ulloa, 1975, 1979)
ILL, extended incision (Marques and Brenda, 1994)	ILL, Greenwald incision (Greenwald, 1987)	ILL, double duck suspension (Cardim et al., 2011)	ILL, italian technique (Sautaché and Bonarrigo, 2004)	ILL, non-scar suspension technique (Echo et al., 2011)
CML, lentoid incision (Greenwald 1985)	CML, triangular incision (Austin, 1994)	CML, rhomboidal incision (Perkins, 2007)	CML, Valentine anguloplasty (Ching and Flowers, 2005)	CML, extended incision (Parsa et al 2010)
CML, lentoid excision for correction of "sad pleats" (Borges, 1989)	VYLA, transverse Y-V (Delerm and Elbaz, 1975)	VYLA, double V-Y (Aiache, 1991)	VYLA, W-shaped incision (Ho, 1994)	VYLA, V-Y in V-Y incision (Mutaf, 2006)

Fig. 6. Summary of all variations of no-filling lip lift. *Red lines* mark the lines of incision, *dotted lines* mark the trajectory of suspension thread, and *compact areas* represent skin excision. CML, corner of the mouth lift; DLL, direct lip lift; ILL, indirect lip lift; V-Y, V-Y plasty; VYLA, V-Y lip augmentation; Y-V, Y-V plasty. (Reprinted with permission *from* Moragas JS, et al. "Non-filling" procedures for lip augmentation: a systematic review of contemporary techniques and their outcomes. J Craniomaxillofac Surg. 2014 Sep;42(6):943-52).

modifications have the advantage of hiding the scar in the buccal vestibule[37] but carry a 4% risk of paresthesia caused by the damage to the branches of infraorbital nerve. Also, theoretically, an intraoral procedure carries the inherent infection risk because of the clean-contaminated nature of the surgical field.[31] In direct lip lift, which has largely fallen out of favor, subtle alterations and visible scarring in the transition between the vermillion and the white skin are likely and it is known as needing a lipstick camouflage.[38]

LIP AUGMENTATION

When volume loss is the main chief complaint, filler and fat grafts may be used or added to the NFPLAs. Moragas and colleagues[39] in another systematic review in

2015 focused on the filling procedures for lip augmentation with the goal of determining the optimal approach. We highly recommend reviewing this comprehensive evidence-based appraisal of the literature, which includes most of the must-know products and techniques in filling procedures for lip augmentation. Facial fillers may be classified into biologic (eg, adipose and collagen) and nonbiologic (eg, silicone). An in-depth discussion of the pros and cons of different products and techniques is beyond the scope of this article. In summary, according to American Society of Aesthetic Plastic Surgeons, hyaluronic acid (HA) seems to be the preferred filler.

A recent meta-analysis has confirmed efficiency of injectable HA in increasing lip fullness for at least 6 months.[40] According to this study, the main adverse effects with the use of HA are tenderness (88.8%), injection site swelling (74.3%), and bruising (39.5%). Rarely, however, more serious reactions including foreign body granulomas (0.6%), herpes labialis (0.6%), and angioedema (0.3%) have occurred. These findings have been consistent with those of Sayan and colleagues[41] who systematically reviewed the adverse reactions associated with laser ablation, administration of fillers, and fat autografting for the rejuvenation of perioral region. They argue that timely recognition of such events and knowledge of their remedies are crucial in safe use of these techniques.[41] To the contrary, a systematic review in 2013 suggested that the uncommon serious reactions (eight events in eight patients of 4605 total patients) were either unrelated (seven events) or probably unrelated (one event) to the procedure.[42] This was consistent with another more recent systematic review, which argues for effectiveness and safety of HA fillers and reports a high patient satisfaction rate.[43] In an evidence-based era, surgeons should develop the ability to critically examine the literature and draw conclusions. We agree with the conclusion drawn by Sayan and colleagues[41] that "training and supervision are essential components of ensuring provision of safe aesthetic treatment, and lack of regulation is a concern."

Regardless of the type of filler, however, knowledge of the precise anatomy of the cutaneous and subcutaneous structures becomes crucial in these scenarios. Vermilion cutaneous junction may be further defined by addition of volume, which is likely to also eliminate perioral rhytides. To restore volume, improve the shape, and achieve lip eversion and pout, fillers or grafts should be injected deep. However, augmenting the more superficial subcutaneous layer is likely to improve the convex shape. The perioral rejuvenation and augmentation is not just limited to the alterations of the upper lip. For instance, the depth of the labiomental crease may be reduced by submentalis fat augmentation to soften the transition line and/or camouflage chin protrusion.[44]

ORTHOGNATHIC SURGERY

The smile width correlates with the maxillary width. Orthognathic smile correction mostly involves Le Fort I osteotomy of the maxilla. In this procedure, maxilla is disengaged from the cephalic end and is moved into a more favorable position in any of the three dimensions to improve facial harmony. Although soft tissue camouflage and orthognathic interventions may significantly improve the smile attractiveness, there is evidence in support of greater and more durable improvements with orthognathic surgeries compared with the former modality. Changes in the maxillary position may also be achieved with other maxillary osteotomies including anterior segmental surgery and segmental Le Fort surgery with differential impaction.[21] A close, often long-term collaboration with an orthodontist trained in the field may be necessary. The work-up of the patient includes clinical photographs and imaging and impressions to develop study casts. A proper data analysis includes formulating a problem list and

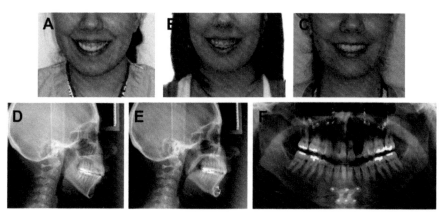

Fig. 7. An example of the effect of orthognathic surgery on smile from preoperative (*A*) and before surgery (*B*) to postoperative (*C*). Imaging shows skeletal changes from preoperative (*D*) to postoperative cephalometry (*E*) and panoramic (*F*) radiograph. (Reprinted with permission *from* Bastidas JA. Surgical Correction of the "Gummy Smile". Oral Maxillofac Surg Clin North Am. 2021 May;33(2):197-209).

a provisional plan.[45] In the digital era, this process may mostly be accomplished electronically, and model surgery may be performed virtually to print the interim and final splints. Traditionally, orthognathic surgeries have been performed after orthodontic intervention. Despite some concerns, however, the surgery-first orthognathic intervention has become a hot topic in maxillofacial surgery[46] with growing evidence supporting its advantages.[47]

Gummy smile caused by VME is an indication for Le Fort corrective surgery. It mainly includes mobilizing the maxilla, removing the excess bony structures from the osteotomized surfaces, and superiorly impacting the maxilla. Le Fort I impaction often includes septoplasty and turbinotomies to make room for adequate impaction (**Fig. 7**). However, a short upper lip challenges the desired outcomes. This method often achieves adequate smile correction unless vertical and horizontal excess are present, in which case multisegmental surgery has yielded successful results.[48] Although an ideal superior repositioning of the maxillary complex may be based on Wolford linear measurements,[49] most surgeons simply use the distance between the mesial incisal edges to lip line at rest. In the past, surgeons used to place a K-wire in the radix for linear measurement reference. This has largely fallen out of favor.[45] Despite the possibility of achieving larger corrections compared with the less invasive camouflages, orthognathic surgery requires higher cost, hospitalization, and a prolonged recovery especially in older adults. Le fort procedures are often associated with significant blood loss and the procedure is preferably done under induced hypotension managed by the anesthesiologist. Patients often experience swelling, pain, midface paresthesia, masticatory and phonation issues, and nasal form alterations. These factors should be considered and discussed with the patient well in advance.

It should be noted that orthognathic surgeries may eliminate or camouflage the chief complaints but may also cause or worsen some other asymmetries of the face. Therefore, touch-up procedures may sometimes be needed to fine-tune the outcomes. Timing of these additional procedures is of utmost importance. Correction of alar base widening, exaggerated labiomental crease, or any other residual deformities after orthognathic surgery results in more predictable outcomes. They should be done either simultaneously at the time of initial orthognathic surgery or as delayed procedures. Alar base widening because of maxillary impaction is often corrected intraoperatively using a variety of methods including the most commonly used alar cinch suture and V-Y closure (**Fig. 8**).[50] In 2014, Khamashta-Ledezma and Naini[45] in a systematic review of the effect of Le Fort I osteotomy with or without cinch sutures and/or V-Y closures on the changes in maxillary incisor exposure and upper lip position, concluded that maxillary advancement increases the soft tissue projection, which is more pronounced at labrale superius compared with pronasale. Anterior nasal spine recontouring, alar base cinch sutures, and V-Y closures seemed to have additive effect, increasing these values. The vertical soft tissue changes were more variable and there were no studies describing the maxillary dental show up to that time. Liu

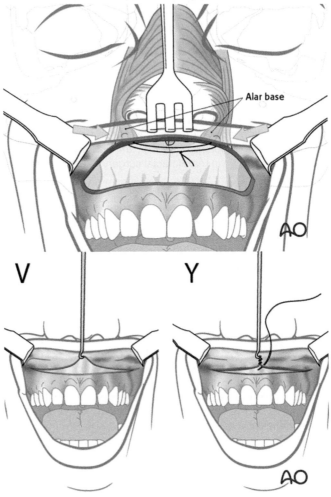

Fig. 8. Schematic presentation of V-Y and alar cinch suture techniques from AO Foundation Web site (https://surgeryreference.aofoundation.org/cmf/trauma/midface/approach/maxillary-vestibular-approach and https://surgeryreference.aofoundation.org/cmf/trauma/midface/approach/maxillary-vestibular-approach).

and colleagues[50] in their systematic review of three studies, including 146 Le Fort I patients, revealed that compared with the classic method, modified transseptal alar base suture and modified reinsertion sutures significantly reduce the postoperative alar base widening (**Fig. 9**). The choice of technique mostly depends on the preference of the OMS.

RHINOPLASTY

Although the use of orthodontics and botulinum toxin injections for the management of gummy smile are well-known and common, rhinoplasty may also significantly improve the nasal and overall facial esthetics in high-smile patients.[51] The upper lip and gum line and the oral and facial anatomic views alter significantly by rhinoplasty. However, surgeons tend to overlook the overall facial harmony assessment in rhinoplasty and only concentrate on the shape and contours of the nose. Few studies have evaluated the effects of rhinoplasty maneuvers on other smile parameters. However, there is growing evidence on the volumetric changes of the upper lip with rhinoplasty and its effect on the static and dynamic changes in the upper lip position.

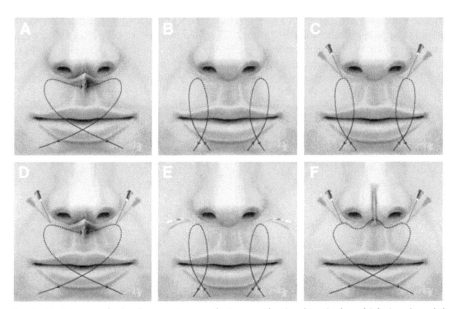

Fig. 9. Variations of alar base suture techniques. Classic alar cinch, which involves (*A*) anchoring the fibroareolar tissues directly under both alae and passing suture through the nasal spine; (*B*) separately anchoring the fibroareolar tissue under both alae intraorally; and (*C*) with the use of hypodermic needles under both alae to accurately identify the nasofacial skinfold, taking a thick suture bite at this point. Modified alar cinch, which involves (*D*) reinsertion using hypodermic needles under both alae and passing the suture through the nasal spine; (*E*) reinsertion using curved needles to anchor the fibroareolar tissue under both alae separately; and (*F*) using hypodermic needles under both alae to accurately identify the nasofacial skinfold, take a thick suture bite at this point, and pass it through the nasal septum. (Reprinted with permission *from* Liu X, et al. Modified versus classic alar base sutures after LeFort I osteotomy: a systematic review. Oral Surg Oral Med Oral Pathol Oral Radiol. 2014 Jan;117(1):37-44).

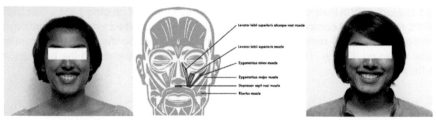

Fig. 10. Correction of gummy smile by botox injection. (left) smile before intervention. (middle) 2.5 units (per 0.1 mL) were injected at 2 sites per side in both overlapping points of the right and left levator labii superioris alaeque nasi, levator labii superioris and zygomaticus minor and levator labii superioris muscle sites. (right) smile 2 weeks after injection of Botox. (*From* Polo M. Botulinum toxin type A (Botox) for the neuromuscular correction of excessive gingival display on smiling (gummy smile). Am J Orthod Dentofacial Orthop. 2008 Feb;133(2):195-203).

Arli et al.[52] found a significant decrease at first and sixth postoperative months in the gingival show in full smile, maxillary incisor-upper lip distance at rest and in full smile, and the interlip distances with rhinoplasty. Brady et al.[53] demonstrated that drooping of the nasal tip is further corrected with the addition of columellar strut grafting to the release of DSN because of the stability it provides. Pi et al.[54] reported a statistically significant decrease in postoperative maxillary incisor show following columella strut, extended spreader graft, and DSN release. They did not see any significant change in maxillary incisor show after nasal spine graft, maxillary augmentation, tip rotation suture, shield graft, columella retraction, or tip suspension suture. Most notably, there was a statistically significant decrease in maxillary incisor show with footplate approximation

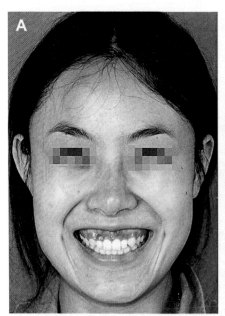
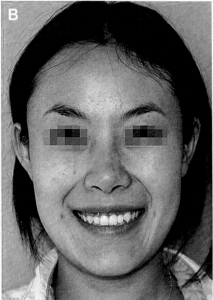

Fig. 11. Patient with severe gummy smile and 1 year following rhinoplasty involving the nasal septum reinforcement. (Reprinted with permission *from* Wei J, et al. Treatment of gummy smile: Nasal septum dysplasia as etiologic factor and therapeutic target. J Plast Reconstr Aesthet Surg. 2015 Oct;68(10):1338-43).

and alar base resection, but this significance was lost when controlling for DSN release. Ho et al.[55] reported the mean change in the upper lip length to be a 1.74% decrease. They found a ~6% decrease in 24 patients (67%), and a ~6% increase in 12 patients (33%) in upper lip length in repose.DSN is a paired muscle contained within the columella and originating from the medial crus of alar cartilage and the caudal of the nasal septum. DSN activation when smiling Disruption of this relationship provides the bases for surgical treatment of tip descent on animation (**Fig. 10**).[52]

NEUROTOXINS

An in-depth discussion about neurotoxins, including Botox, could be easily found on several scientific forums. We recommend the textbook *Facial Cosmetic Surgery* by Niamtu[54] for further reading.

In brief, in patients with gummy smile and hyperactive nasal tip, DSN paralysis using botulinum toxin injections is an alternative to surgical resection without rhinoplasty (**Fig. 11**).[55] This results in the upturn of the nasal tip and prevents depression of the tip during speaking and smiling. An injection of two Botox units just below each side of the columella tends to be adequate for optimal results. Because the injection may contribute to lip ptosis, DSN paralysis is likely to result in worsening of a long upper lip or low vermilion show. Niamtu has explained implementing a "conservative progression of injections" where two injections of 2.5 Botox units each are done lateral to each alar base and the patient is assessed in 7 to 10 days. If adequate results are achieved at this point, no further intervention is indicated. Otherwise the same injection sequence and dose are repeated.[54]

Nasolabial folds extend from the nostrils to the lateral perioral region and play an important role in overall esthetics and youthfulness of the midface. Although some clinicians inject both LLSAN at the level of the bony lateral nasal rim to soften this fold, the relaxation is believed to be minimal and may cause dysfunctional animation or lip elongation. Snider and colleagues[56] have introduced a better injection site based on a cadaver study to avoid changing upper lip position. This point is located around 8.4 mm inferior and 4.6 mm medial to the medial canthus, far away from the LLS and targets the superior aspect of the LLSAN. Additionally, injection into this alternative site may soften the effect of the LLSAN on the lateral nasal sidewall rhytids, also known as "bunny lines."[56]

OTHER INTERVENTIONS

Several other interventions exist for the alteration, augmentation, and/or correction of the smile asymmetries. Literature, including several issues of the Clinics, have explored these venues in detail. Fillers and especially fat autografts have also gained popularity in redefining, volumization, and rejuvenation of the lips and improving the smile esthetics as stand-alone procedures or as additions to rhinoplasty and/or orthognathic surgeries.[50] Smile asymmetries caused by facial nerve palsies or cleft lip and/or palate need a separate comprehensive review.

CLINICS CARE POINTS

---

deferentiation of the etiology of gummy smile is crucial to assure proper management:

- VME is usually corrected with LeFort I impation.
- Short crown maybe corrected with gingivoplasty.

- hyperactive lip may be corrected with surgical or chemical lysis.

REFERENCE

1. Sabri R. The eight components of a balanced smile. J Clin Orthod 2005;39(3): 155–67.
2. Khambay BS, Lowney CJ, Hsung TC, et al. Fluctuating asymmetry of dynamic smiles in normal individuals. Int J Oral Maxillofac Surg 2019;48(10):1372–9.
3. Rostami S, Kang B, Tufekci E, et al. Recognition of the asymmetrical smile: a comparison of orthodontists, oral and maxillofacial surgeons, and laypersons. J Oral Maxillofac Surg 2020;78(2):275–83.
4. Ding A. The ideal lips: lessons learnt from the literature. Aesthetic Plast Surg 2021;45(4):1520–30.
5. Harris R, Nagarkar P, Amirlak B. Varied definitions of nasolabial angle: searching for consensus among rhinoplasty surgeons and an algorithm for selecting the ideal method. Plast Reconstr Surg Glob open 2016;4(6):e752.
6. Brown M, Guyuron B. Redefining the ideal nasolabial angle: Part 2. Expert analysis. Plast Reconstr Surg 2013;132(2):221e–5e.
7. Armijo BS, Brown M, Guyuron B. Defining the ideal nasolabial angle. Plast Reconstr Surg 2012;129(3):759–64.
8. Understanding the perioral anatomy. Plast Surg Nurs 2016;36(1):E1.
9. Shim K-S, Hu K-S, Kwak H-H, et al. An anatomical study of the insertion of the zygomaticus major muscle in humans focused on the muscle arrangement at the corner of the mouth. Plast Reconstr Surg 2008;121(2):466–73.
10. Elvan Ö, Bobus Örs A, Tezer MS. Anatomical evaluation of zygomaticus major muscle with relation to orbicularis oculi muscle and parotid duct. J Craniofac Surg 2020;31(6):1844–7.
11. Rubin LR. The anatomy of a smile: its importance in the treatment of facial paralysis. Plast Reconstr Surg 1974;53(4):384–7.
12. Rubin LR, Mishriki Y, Lee G. Anatomy of the nasolabial fold: the keystone of the smiling mechanism. Plast Reconstr Surg 1989;83(1):1–10.
13. Bao S, Zhou C, Li S, et al. A new simple technique for making facial dimples. Aesthetic Plast Surg 2007;31(4):380–3.
14. Ewart CJ, Jaworski NB, Rekito AJ, et al. Levator anguli oris: a cadaver study implicating its role in perioral rejuvenation. Ann Plast Surg 2005;54(3):260–3.
15. Sarver DM, Ackerman MB. Dynamic smile visualization and quantification: Part 2. Smile analysis and treatment strategies. Am J Orthod Dentofacial Orthop 2003; 124(2):116–27.
16. Sawyer AR, See M, Nduka C. Quantitative analysis of normal smile with 3D stereophotogrammetry: an aid to facial reanimation. J Plast Reconstr Aesthet Surg 2010;63(1):65–72.
17. Garber DA, Salama MA. The aesthetic smile: diagnosis and treatment. Periodontol 2000 1996;11:18–28.
18. Ebrahimi A, Nejadsarvari N, Motamedi MH, et al. Anatomic variations found on dissection of depressor septi nasi muscles in cadavers. Arch Facial Plast Surg 2012;14(1):31–3.
19. Sinno S, Chang JB, Saadeh PB, et al. Anatomy and surgical treatment of the depressor septi nasi muscle: a systematic review. Plast Reconstr Surg 2015; 135(5):838e–48e.

20. Benson KJ, Laskin DM. Upper lip asymmetry in adults during smiling. J Oral Maxillofac Surg 2001;59(4):396–8.
21. Reis GM, de Freitas DS, Oliveira RC, et al. Smile attractiveness in class III patients after orthodontic camouflage or orthognathic surgery. Clin Oral Investig 2021;25(12):6791–7.
22. Gowd S, Shankar T, Chatterjee S, et al. Gingival zenith positions and levels of maxillary anterior dentition in cases of bimaxillary protrusion: a morphometric analysis. J Contemp Dent Pract 2017;18(8):700–4.
23. Simon Z, Rosenblatt A. Challenges in achieving gingival harmony. J Calif Dental Assoc 2010;38 8:583–90.
24. Tarnow DP, Magner AW, Fletcher P. The effect of the distance from the contact point to the crest of bone on the presence or absence of the interproximal dental papilla. J Periodontol 1992;63(12):995–6.
25. Roccuzzo M, Roccuzzo A, Ramanuskaite A. Papilla height in relation to the distance between bone crest and interproximal contact point at single-tooth implants: a systematic review. Clin Oral Implants Res 2018;29(Suppl 15):50–61.
26. Ramanauskaite A, Roccuzzo A, Schwarz F. A systematic review on the influence of the horizontal distance between two adjacent implants inserted in the anterior maxilla on the inter-implant mucosa fill. Clin Oral Implants Res 2018;29(Suppl 15): 62–70.
27. Jung RE, Heitz-Mayfield L, Schwarz F. Evidence-based knowledge on the aesthetics and maintenance of peri-implant soft tissues: Osteology Foundation Consensus Report Part 3-Aesthetics of peri-implant soft tissues. Clin Oral Implants Res 2018;29(Suppl 15):14–7.
28. Schwarz F, Giannobile WV, Jung RE. Evidence-based knowledge on the aesthetics and maintenance of peri-implant soft tissues: Osteology Foundation Consensus Report Part 2-Effects of hard tissue augmentation procedures on the maintenance of peri-implant tissues. Clin Oral Implants Res 2018;29(Suppl 15):11–3.
29. Yamin F, McAuliffe PB, Vasilakis V. Aesthetic surgical enhancement of the upper lip: a comprehensive literature review. Aesthetic Plast Surg 2021;45(1):173–80.
30. Salibian AA, Bluebond-Langner R. Lip lift. Facial Plast Surg Clin North Am 2019; 27(2):261–6.
31. Moragas JS, Vercruysse HJ, Mommaerts MY. Non-filling" procedures for lip augmentation: a systematic review of contemporary techniques and their outcomes. J Craniomaxillofac Surg 2014;42(6):943–52.
32. DeJoseph LM, Agarwal A, Greco TM. Lip augmentation. Facial Plast Surg Clin North Am 2018;26(2):193–203.
33. Waldman SR. The subnasal lift. Facial Plast Surg Clin North Am 2007;15(4): 513–6, viii.
34. Echo A, Momoh AO, Yuksel E. The no-scar lip-lift: upper lip suspension technique. Aesthetic Plast Surg 2011;35(4):617–23.
35. Cardim VLN, Silva AdS, Salomons RL, et al. Double duck" nasolabial lifting. Revista Brasileira de Cirurgia Plástica 2011;26:466–71.
36. Mommaerts MY, Blythe JN. Rejuvenation of the ageing upper lip and nose with suspension lifting. J Cranio-Maxillofacial Surg 2016;44(9):1123–5.
37. Obradovic B, Obradovic M. Triple V-Y vermilion augmentation of the upper lip. J Craniofac Surg 2015;26(8):e736–8.
38. Guerrissi JO. Surgical treatment of the senile upper lip. Plast Reconstr Surg 2000; 106(4):938–40.

39. San Miguel Moragas J, Reddy RR, Hernández Alfaro F, et al. Systematic review of "filling" procedures for lip augmentation regarding types of material, outcomes and complications. J Craniomaxillofac Surg 2015;43(6):883–906.

40. Czumbel LM, Farkasdi S, Gede N, et al. Hyaluronic acid is an effective dermal filler for lip augmentation: a meta-analysis. Front Surg 2021;8:681028.

41. Sayan A, Gonen ZB, Ilankovan V. Adverse reactions associated with perioral rejuvenation using laser, fat and hyaluronic acid: systematic review. Br J Oral Maxillofac Surg 2021;59(9):1005–12.

42. Cohen JL, Dayan SH, Brandt FS, et al. Systematic review of clinical trials of small- and large-gel-particle hyaluronic acid injectable fillers for aesthetic soft tissue augmentation. Dermatol Surg 2013;39(2):205–31.

43. Stojanovič L, Majdič N. Effectiveness and safety of hyaluronic acid fillers used to enhance overall lip fullness: a systematic review of clinical studies. J Cosmet Dermatol 2019;18(2):436–43.

44. Rohrich RJ, Pessa JE. The anatomy and clinical implications of perioral submuscular fat. Plast Reconstr Surg 2009;124(1):266–71.

45. Khamashta-Ledezma L, Naini FB. Systematic review of changes in maxillary incisor exposure and upper lip position with Le Fort I type osteotomies with or without cinch sutures and/or VY closures. Int J Oral Maxillofac Surg 2014;43(1):46-61.

46. Choi JW, Lee JY. Current concept of the surgery-first orthognathic approach. Arch Plast Surg 2021;48(2):199–207.

47. Choi JW, Park H, Kwon SM, et al. Surgery-first orthognathic approach for the correction of facial asymmetry. J Craniomaxillofac Surg 2021;49(6):435–42.

48. Nishiyama A, Ibaragi S, Yoshioka N, et al. A case of maxillary protrusion and gummy smile treated by multi-segmental horseshoe Le Fort I osteotomy. Int J Oral Maxillofac Surg 2017;46:327.

49. Fish LC, Wolford LM, Epker BN. Surgical-orthodontic correction of vertical maxillary excess. Am J Orthod 1978;73(3):241–57.

50. Liu X, Zhu S, Hu J. Modified versus classic alar base sutures after LeFort I osteotomy: a systematic review. Oral Surg Oral Med Oral Pathol Oral Radiol 2014;117(1):37-44.

51. Rohrich RJ, Ahmad J. A practical approach to rhinoplasty. Plast Reconstr Surg 2016;137(4):725e–46e.

52. Arli C, Bilgic F, Kaya A, et al. Effects of rhinoplasty on smile esthetic and gingival appearance. J Craniofac Surg 2020;31(3):689–91.

53. Brady C, Berwick D, Uppal R. Tip droop prevention in rhinoplasty: dynamic effect of strut graft on smiling versus depressor muscle release. Plast Reconstr Surg Glob Open 2021;9(4):e3462.

54. Niamtu J. Cosmetic facial surgery. Second edition. Edinburgh: Elsevier; 2018.

55. Benlier E, Balta S, Tas S. Depressor septi nasi modifications in rhinoplasty: a review of anatomy and surgical techniques. Facial Plast Surg 2014;30(4):471–6.

56. Snider CC, Amalfi AN, Hutchinson LE, et al. New insights into the anatomy of the midface musculature and its implications on the nasolabial fold. Aesthetic Plast Surg 2017;41(5):1083–90.

Crown Lengthening Techniques and Modifications to Treat Excessive Gingival Display

Maziar Shahzad Dowlatshahi, DDS, MSc[a],*,
Ghazal Anoosh, DDS, MSc[b], Jorge Alania, DDS[c],
Jessica M. Latimer, DDS[d]

KEYWORDS

- Crown lengthening • Gingivoplasty • Esthetics • Dental • Periodontium

KEY POINTS

- Aesthetic crown lengthening relies on harmonious integration of the facial, dental, and periodontal components.
- Selection of surgical techniques for clinical crown lengthening is diagnosis-dependent.
- Maintenance of the supracrestal tissue attachment and keratinized gingiva are essential biologic requirements for successful clinical outcomes.

INTRODUCTION

A *smile* is a human facial expression composed of the spatial relationships of the face, lips, and teeth.[1] Although a smile may convey different emotions depending on the socio-cultural context, in North America, it is generally associated with positive emotional states such as happiness, pleasure, and amusement. An individual may be perceived as more attractive, friendly, intelligent, trustworthy, self-confident, or even successful based on their smile.[2–4]

In a landmark study of body image, Berscheid and colleagues[5] reported that most Americans found dental appearance significant in social interactions. Moreover, in a 2013 survey conducted by the American Academy of Cosmetic Dentistry, the most common reason patients cited for pursuing cosmetic dental treatment was to improve physical attractiveness and self-esteem.

[a] Private Practice, 8500 Leslie Street, Suite 220, Toronto, Ontario, Canada; [b] Department of Periodontics, Faculty of Dentistry, Tehran Medical Sciences, Islamic Azad University, Tehran, Iran; [c] Private Practice, Victor Maurtua Avenue 140, Office 407, San Isidro, Lima, Peru; [d] Department of Oral Medicine, Infection, and Immunity, Harvard School of Dental Medicine, 188 Longwood Avenue, Boston, MA 02115, USA
* Corresponding author.
E-mail address: dowlatshahimsh@gmail.com

Dent Clin N Am 66 (2022) 361–372
https://doi.org/10.1016/j.cden.2022.03.002
0011-8532/22/© 2022 Elsevier Inc. All rights reserved.

Excessive gingival display (or gummy smile) is a prevalent aesthetic problem in dentistry described by the American Academy of Periodontology as a mucogingival deformity around teeth.[6] Approximately 10% of the population between the ages of 20 and 30 are affected and it is more common in women than in men.[7,8] Etiologic factors for this clinical presentation may include gingival enlargement, altered passive eruption, vertical maxillary excess, short lip length, lip hypermobility, or various combinations of these conditions.[9,10] When planning treatment for aesthetically demanding cases, smile design cannot be isolated from a comprehensive approach to patient care. This entails coordinated management of the health and appearance of the teeth, periodontium, orofacial muscles, underlying skeletal structures, and joints. A well-developed and algorithmic evaluation is needed for predictable diagnosis and treatment.

AESTHETIC CONSIDERATIONS
Facial Components

Aesthetic smile design requires the integration of the facial, dental, and periodontal features of a patient. The facial composition includes the hard and soft tissues of the face.[11] The dental composition includes the teeth and their relationship with the periodontal tissues. Unless there is an obvious discrepancy in the facial features, we often restrict our smile design to the dental composition only. The primary facial component that must be considered during the initial evaluation is the lip line, which may be defined as the position of the inferior border of the upper lip when smiling. The position of the lip line when smiling determines the display of the teeth and/or gingiva; the smile line can be classified into 3 major categories[7]:

- High: 100% of the cervicoincisal length of the maxillary incisors are exposed and a contiguous band of gingiva is displayed
- Average: 75% to 100% of the maxillary incisors and only the interdental papillae are exposed
- Low: less than 75% of the cervicoincisal length of the maxillary incisors are exposed

In the original comparative study conducted by Tjan and colleagues,[7] a normal smile line was found in 313 (68.94%) of 454 subjects, whereas 93 subjects (20.48%) were categorized as having an average smile line and a high smile line was found in 48 subjects (10.57%), thus representing the least common smile type. Normal gingival display is typically 1 to 2 mm and exposure that exceeds 3 mm is considered unaesthetic.[12,13]

Dental Components

The dental component should be well balanced with the face as well as follow ideal proportions. Important aspects of the dental component, such as the incisal edge position, smile arc, axial inclination, interdental contact position, incisal embrasures, shape, color, symmetry, and overall balance should be considered. These characteristics also may be influenced by the patient's sex, personality, and age. More details regarding smile design considerations for the teeth are provided in chapters 1, 11, and 12. Otherwise, the primary dental consideration in aesthetic crown lengthening is tooth dimension of the maxillary anterior teeth. The ideal width-to-length ratio of the central incisors is 85% and the ideal ratio is 80% for the lateral incisors and canines.[14] Typically, cases indicated for aesthetic crown lengthening present with teeth that appear to be square in form due to a normal width of the teeth accompanied by a deficiency in the length of the clinical crowns.

Periodontal Components

Before the initiation of any treatment, gingival health is of paramount importance and a prerequisite factor.[15] Inflammation may be a primary cause of gingival hyperplasia, and resolution following therapy can improve the aesthetic appearance of the gingiva. The gingival tissues frame the teeth as they influence the size and shape of the clinical crown. Aesthetic guidelines for key features of the gingival architecture are outlined here:

1. Gingival margins[16]
   - Should be symmetric for the maxillary central incisors.
   - The gingival margins of the maxillary incisors and canines should be on the same plane.
   - The gingival margin level of the maxillary laterals are ideally located 0.5 to 2 mm incisal to the central incisors and canine teeth.
2. Gingival shape
   - A half circular shape for the mandibular incisors and the maxillary laterals is ideal.
   - An elliptical shape is recommended for the maxillary centrals and canines.
3. Gingival zenith[17]
   - Located 1 mm distal to the long axis of the maxillary centrals.
   - Located 0.4 mm distal to the long axis of the maxillary lateral incisors.
   - Coincides with the long axis of the maxillary canines.
4. Interdental papillae[18]
   - The interdental papillae should fill the interproximal space between the gingiva and the contact area.
   - The distance from the contact point to the crest of bone should be 5 mm or less to accomplish complete papilla fill.
   - If the crest to contact distance is 6 mm, the papilla is present 56% of the time.
   - If the distance is >7 mm or more, the papilla is present 27% of the time.

TREATMENT PLANNING

The purpose of surgical crown lengthening is to increase the extent of the supragingival tooth structure. Various therapeutic approaches may be considered to correct excessive gingival display and technique selection is diagnosis-dependent. If excessive gingival display occurs when smiling, the length and activity of the upper lip must first be considered. The lip length is measured from the base of the nose to the wet border of the maxillary lip at rest, which is usually 20 to 22 mm in female patients and 22 to 24 mm in male patients.[8] If the etiology of excessive gingival display is attributed to a short lip or lip hyperactivity, no clinical crown lengthening (CCL) treatment is indicated. Lip repositioning, augmentation, and lip lift techniques can be reviewed in chapters 4, 8, and 9.

Evaluation of the dentogingival features are considered next. The positions of the gingival margin, cementoenamel junction (CEJ), and osseous crest should be examined. This necessitates an understanding of the active and passive phases of tooth eruption. Active eruption ceases when the teeth come into contact with the opposing dentition. Passive eruption is characterized by the apical migration of the epithelial attachment to expose the anatomic crown. The delay or failure of passive eruption results in short clinical crowns, in which the gingival margin is positioned coronal to the CEJ; this condition is termed altered passive eruption (APE). APE is a common etiologic component of excessive gingival display; a 12.1% incidence of APE was reported in a study of 1025 patients with a mean age of 24.2 ± 6.2 years.[19] Other factors that can contribute to excessive gingival display include vertical maxillary excess, in which the gingival display is ≥ 8 mm, anterior overeruption, and gingival enlargement. Garber and Salama[20] presented a classification system for excessive gingival display and their proposed treatments:

- Degree I with 2 to 4 mm of the gingival display. Recommended treatment is orthodontic intrusion alone, orthodontics, crown lengthening, or crown lengthening followed by restorations.
- Degree II with 4 to 8 mm of the gingival display. Recommended treatment is crown lengthening and restorations or orthognathic surgery, depending on the crown root ratio.
- Degree III with ≥ 8 mm of the gingival display. Recommended treatment is orthognathic surgery with or without crown lengthening and restorative treatment.

Regarding overall treatment sequence, cause-related therapy should be performed during phase I. In cases of periodontal disease and inflammation without gingival overgrowth, periodontal treatment will resolve the gingival swelling by removing irritating local factors.[21] Endodontic treatments should be rendered if indicated, then periodontal surgery in cases of periodontitis. Finally, crown lengthening procedures can be performed after stable, periodontal health is achieved.

ANATOMIC CONSIDERATIONS

Successful CCL surgery relies on 2 key anatomic factors: establishment of the supracrestal tissue attachment (SCTA) and maintenance of an adequate width (≥ 2 mm) of keratinized gingiva (KG).[21–23] The SCTA, previously known as the biologic width, is defined as the dimension of healthy gingival tissue that exists coronally to the alveolar bone, involving the sum of the junctional epithelium and the connective tissue dimensions.[24–26] In the classic study by Gargiulo and colleagues,[26] the average dimensions of the epithelial attachment and connective tissue were 0.97 and 1.07, respectively, resulting in an average biologic width or SCTA of 2.04 mm. Although a 2-mm mean dimension of the SCTA has been validated by numerous studies involving clinical, radiographic, and/or histologic evaluation, significant intra-individual and inter-individual variance exist, ranging from 0.2 to 6.73 mm.[27]

A minimum of 3 mm of space between the restorative margin and alveolar bone crest has been determined to be adequate for periodontal health, allowing 2 mm of space for the SCTA and 1 mm for the sulcus depth.[23,28] If impingement of the SCTA occurs, reestablishment of the original dimension will occur through bone resorption or chronic gingival inflammation around the tooth. Subsequently, consequences such as gingival enlargement, gingival recession, and periodontal pocket formation may follow.[29,30] Overall, the SCTA serves as a barrier against microbial entry in the periodontium and is a fundamental aspect of the periodontal attachment apparatus.[29] It should always be measured before any CCL surgeries and maintained during restorative procedures to preserve periodontal health.[23]

Bone sounding (BS), also referred to as transgingival probing, was first recommended in 1976 by Greenberg and colleagues[31] to estimate the level of the osseous crest. The dimension of the SCTA can be calculated by subtracting the probing depth of the sulcus from the measurement obtained by BS. Although intraoperative bone level measurements performed with direct vision are the most accurate, BS offers a minimally invasive approach for measuring the facial osseous-gingival tissue relationship (FOGTR) with comparable accuracy.[32] The FOGTR may be difficult to evaluate in patients with APE because the buccal bone crest at the level of or coronal to the CEJ can prevent its detection, even in the presence of a pseudopocket. Moreover, when the facial gingiva is tightly attached to the tooth by the junctional epithelium in health, BS can also become more difficult. The patient should be thoroughly anesthetized before BS.

Based on the amount of KG and distance of the crestal bone to the CEJ or future restorative margin, 4 possible clinical situations were described by Coslet and colleagues.[33] Type I cases involve adequate KG ($\geq$2 mm) whereas Type II cases present with inadequate KG (<2 mm).[33] Both case types can be further divided into subgroups A and B, in which the distance of the CEJ to the osseous crest is $\geq$2 mm or <2 mm, respectively. Treatment indications depend on the case classification[33]:

- Type IA: adequate KG ($\geq$2 mm) and $\geq$2 mm CEJ-osseous crest
  - Recommended treatment: gingivectomy only
- Type IB: adequate KG ($\geq$2 mm) and <2 mm CEJ-osseous crest
  - Recommended treatment: gingivectomy or internal beveled incision with flap repositioned with osseous resection
- Type IIA: inadequate KG (<2 mm) and $\geq$2 mm CEJ-osseous crest
  - Recommended treatment: apically positioned flap; no osseous recontouring
- Type IIA: inadequate KG (<2 mm) and <2 mm CEJ-osseous crest
  - Recommended treatment: apically positioned flap with osseous resection

Before surgery, the dimensions of the SCTA should be measured for each tooth. The CEJ provides a reference point for placement of an incision that follows the aesthetic smile line, provided that at least 2 mm of KG remains on the facial aspect of the teeth. It is vital to design and prepare a provisional or mock-up crowns to act as an aesthetic surgical template that dictates the desired length, width, and shape of the teeth involved; this guide may be used in diagnosis, treatment planning, and surgery.[34] The surgical template guides the placement of the buccal incisions according to the aesthetic smile design. After flap reflection, the template provides reference so that the margin of the future clinical crown and the osseous crest levels can be established and maintained through the bone-contouring process.

Special considerations accompany each case type.[33] In type IA cases, the provisional restoration may be placed immediately after gingivectomy provided there is adequate hemostasis.

In type 1B cases, it is recommended to raise a full-thickness flap on the facial and a partial-thickness on the interdental papillae to leave it intact without any vertical releasing incisions or a palatal flap. Based on the distance of the CEJ to the osseous crest distance and the dimensions of the SCTA, osseous resection may be performed. It is recommended to remove the bone only at the mid-facial area, unless the SCTA indicates that it is necessary to remove bone in interdental areas, blending it toward the mesiofacial and distofacial line angles to establish the SCTA. Precise adaptation of the interdental papillae is necessary to minimize the risk of increased gingival embrasure spaces. This will promote maximum preservation of the interdental soft tissue and gingival margin configuration.[35] End-cutting burs and round diamond burs may be used in this procedure. The buccal flap is replaced at the level of the CEJ, surgical guide, printed template, or slightly above it. Because more significant gingival proliferation occurs when the flap margin is positioned closer to the bone crest, the flap should be placed coronally rather than apically to maximize tissue preservation and gingival margin stability and predictability during subsequent healing and maturation. Vertical mattress sutures can be used to secure the flap slightly coronally and periosteal sutures that will apically position the flap and place the gingival margin close to the bone crest should be avoided.[36]

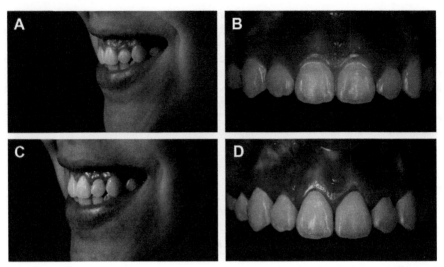

Fig. 1. Clinical case example #1 demonstrating excessive gingival display due to APE. (*A*) Preoperative extraoral profile. (*B*) Preoperative intraoral photos. (*C*) Postoperative extraoral profile. (*D*) Postoperative intraoral photos at 8 weeks healing.

Secondary surgery may be needed to finalize the exact position of the gingival margin after 6 to 12 weeks.

A subsequent gingivectomy procedure may be performed, accompanied by placement of the provisional restorations.

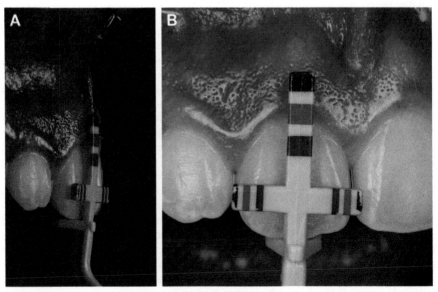

Fig. 2. Preoperative intraoral evaluation of tooth #8 using a Chu gauge in (*A*) profile and in a (*B*) frontal view to assess tooth proportions and determine the new position of the alveolar bone required for predictable, esthetic correction.

Type II cases involve an insufficient amount of KG, an apically displaced flap is recommended to preserve the KG while still establishing an ideal position of the margin. **Figs. 1–5.**

Postoperative Considerations

The healing time and stability of the surgically established gingival margin positions are important factors that can impact the final treatment outcome, especially if the teeth are to be restored. Improper planning may lead to uneven gingival margins, loss of interdental papillae, or recession. Functional arrangement and collagenous maturation of the gingival connective tissue occurs 3 to 5 weeks after gingivectomy.[37] If flap reflection and bone exposure are also involved, at least 8 to 12 weeks healing time is necessary. Further, if ostectomy is performed, at least 6 months is required for hard and soft tissue stabilization.[38,39]

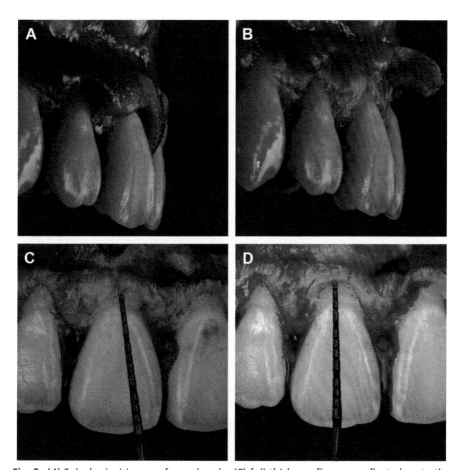

Fig. 3. (A) Sulcular incisions performed and a (B) full-thickness flap was reflected up to the mucogingival junction to maintain the position at the same level after gingivectomy. Dissection past the mucogingival junction should be avoided to prevent mobility. (C) Preoperatively, the alveolar crest was measured at a distance of 1 mm apical to the CEJ of tooth #8. (D) After ostectomy, the new position of the alveolar crest was established 3 mm apical to the CEJ.

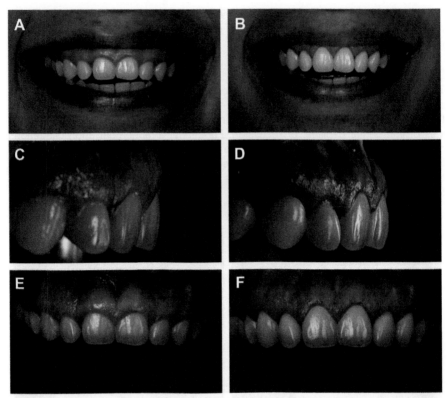

Fig. 4. Clinical case example #2 of a patient with excessive gingival display and broad smile showing maxillary teeth from #3 to 14. Extraoral (*A*) preoperative and (*B*) postoperative frontal photos, intraoral (*C*) preoperative and (*D*) postoperative profile photos, and intraoral (*E*) preoperative and (*F*) postoperative frontal photos. Postoperative photos were taken at 12 weeks of healing. CCL was performed with ostectomy and apically positioned flap.

Postoperatively, the supracrestal gingival tissues remodel and mature to regain their original dimension. Pontoriero and Carnevale[40] demonstrated that after use of an apically positioned flap and osseous resection, the marginal gingival tissue proliferates in a coronal direction; at 1 year, they observed reductions in clinical crown length of 0.5 ± 0.6 mm at interproximal sites and 1.2 ± 0.7 mm at buccal/lingual sites; however in their study, the flaps were positioned at or apical to the osseous crest. Deas and colleagues[38] reported that significant tissue rebound can occur when the flap margin is sutured too close (>1 mm) to the osseous crest. Lanning and colleagues[41] presented a protocol to measure the SCTA preoperatively and determine the amount of osseous resection required based on the dimensions of the SCTA and planned position of the future restorative margin; with this approach, most (90%) sites required bone removal of at least 3 mm. The gingival margin positions were found to be stable at 3 months and remained unchanged for the remainder of the 6-month observation period.

DISCUSSION

For dentists, aesthetics is one of the ultimate goals of the clinical treatment delivered. For patients, the appearance of their smile can have a significant impact on self-

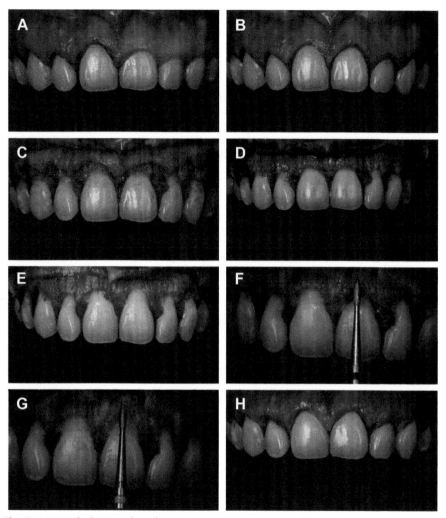

Fig. 5. Intraoral photos taken during surgery demonstrating (*A*) initial gingivectomy with (*B*) internal bevel incisions to teeth #4 and 13 to facilitate surgical access and (*C*) expose maxillary buccal exostoses. (*D*) Ostectomy was performed accompanied by osteoplasty using a flame-shaped diamond bur on low rotation in (*E*) and (*F*) fine and (*G*) extra-fine. (*H*) The flap was sutured with polydioxanone monofilament absorbable 6/0 DS-15 to the ideal position.

esteem and perception by others. An organized, systematic, and multidisciplinary approach is required to treat aesthetic concerns with predictable, stable results. Different etiologic factors must be considered and an accurate diagnosis is necessary to provide an appropriate treatment plan.

The main techniques used for surgical crown lengthening are the following:

- External bevel gingivectomy
- Internal bevel incision with or without bone resection
- Apically positioned flap with or without bone resection
- Combined technique (surgical and orthodontic)

The key to successful treatment is selecting the appropriate techniques to correct the anatomic problems, maintain the biologic width, and achieve the visualized final aesthetic result.

SUMMARY

Proper evaluation, diagnosis, treatment planning, and surgical technique will promote an optimal and stable aesthetic outcome. Biologic requirements of the anatomic structures must be satisfied. Finally, although the correction of the excessive gingival display can dramatically enhance smile aesthetics, it can also provide great satisfaction to the patient and positively impact their quality of life.

CLINICS CARE POINTS

- Assessment of the etiology of the excessive gingival display is mandatory, as technique selection for CCL is diagnosis-dependent.
- Accurate preoperative measurements of the SCTA must be obtained for each tooth to determine the amount of osseous resection needed, if any.
- A surgical template, provisional restorations, or mock-up crowns should be used intraoperatively as reference points to establish the new FOGTR.
- Tissue rebound can occur when the flap margins are sutured too close to the alveolar bone crest.
- Results are stabilized after 6 months.

DISCLOSURE

The authors have nothing to disclose.

REFERENCES

1. Bhuvaneswaran M. Principles of smile design. J Conserv Dent 2010;13(4): 225–32.
2. Kerosuo H, Hausen H, Laine T, et al. The influence of incisal malocclusion on the social attractiveness of young adults in Finland. Eur J Orthod 1995;17(6):505–12.
3. Flores-Mir C, Silva E, Barriga MI, et al. Lay person's perception of smile aesthetics in dental and facial views. J Orthod 2004;31(3):204–9 ; discussion 201.
4. Malkinson S, Waldrop TC, Gunsolley JC, et al. The effect of esthetic crown lengthening on perceptions of a patient's attractiveness, friendliness, trustworthiness, intelligence, and self-confidence. J Periodontol 2013;84(8):1126–33.
5. Berscheid E, Walster E, Bohrnstedt G. The happy American body: a survey report. Psychol Today 1973;7:119–31.
6. Armitage GC. Development of a classification system for periodontal diseases and conditions. Ann Periodontol 1999;4(1):1–6.
7. Tjan AH, Miller GD, The JG. Some esthetic factors in a smile. J Prosthet Dent 1984;51(1):24–8.
8. Peck S, Peck L, Kataja M. The gingival smile line. Angle Orthod 1992;62(2): 91–100, discussion 101-2.
9. Dolt AH 3rd, Robbins JW. Altered passive eruption: an etiology of short clinical crowns. Quintessence Int 1997;28(6):363–72.

10. Levine RA, McGuire M. The diagnosis and treatment of the gummy smile. Compend Contin Educ Dent 1997;18(8):757–62, 764; quiz 766.
11. Kokich VO Jr, Kiyak HA, Shapiro PA. Comparing the perception of dentists and lay people to altered dental esthetics. J Esthet Dent 1999;11(6):311–24.
12. Kokich VO, Kokich VG, Kiyak HA. Perceptions of dental professionals and laypersons to altered dental esthetics: asymmetric and symmetric situations. Am J Orthod Dentofacial Orthop 2006;130(2):141–51.
13. Levin EI. Dental esthetics and the golden proportion. J Prosthet Dent 1978;40(3): 244–52.
14. Álvarez-Álvarez L, Orozco-Varo A, Arroyo-Cruz G, et al. Width/length ratio in maxillary anterior teeth. Comparative study of esthetic preferences among professionals and laypersons. J Prosthodont 2019;28(4):416–20.
15. Chiche GJ, Pinault A. Smile rejuvenation: a methodic approach. Pract Periodontics Aesthet Dent 1993;5(3):37–44 ; quiz 44.
16. Machado AW. 10 commandments of smile esthetics. Dental Press J Orthod 2014; 19(4):136–57.
17. Chu SJ, Tan JH, Stappert CF, et al. Gingival zenith positions and levels of the maxillary anterior dentition. J Esthet Restor Dent 2009;21(2):113–20.
18. Tarnow DP, Magner AW, Fletcher P. The effect of the distance from the contact point to the crest of bone on the presence or absence of the interproximal dental papilla. J Periodontol 1992;63(12):995–6.
19. Volchansky A, Cleaton-jones P. Delayed passive eruption - A predisposing factor to Vincent's infection. J. Dent. Assoc. S. Afr. 1974;29:291–4.
20. Garber DA, Salama MA. The aesthetic smile: diagnosis and treatment. Periodontol 2000;11:18–28. Jun 1996.
21. Ong M, Tseng S, Wang H. Crown lengthening revisited. Clin Adv Periodontics 2017;1(3):233–9.
22. Maynard JG Jr, Wilson RD. Physiologic dimensions of the periodontium significant to the restorative dentist. J Periodontol 1979;50(4):170–4.
23. Nevins M, Skurow HM. The intracrevicular restorative margin, the biologic width, and the maintenance of the gingival margin. Int J Periodontics Restorative Dent 1984;4(3):30–49.
24. Vacek JS, Gher ME, Assad DA, et al. The dimensions of the human dentogingival junction. Int J Periodontics Restorative Dent 1994;14(2):154–65.
25. Jepsen S, Caton JG, Albandar JM, et al. Periodontal manifestations of systemic diseases and developmental and acquired conditions: consensus report of workgroup 3 of the 2017 world workshop on the classification of periodontal and peri-implant diseases and conditions. J Periodontol 2018;89(Suppl 1):S237–48.
26. Gargiulo A, Wentz FM, Orban B. Dimensions and relations of the dentogingival junction in humans. J Periodontol 1961;32:261–7.
27. Schmidt JC, Sahrmann P, Weiger R, et al. Biologic width dimensions–a systematic review. J Clin Periodontol 2013;40(5):493–504.
28. Block PL. Restorative margins and periodontal health: a new look at an old perspective. J Prosthet Dent 1987;57(6):683–9.
29. Carvalho BAS, Duarte CAB, Silva JF, et al. Clinical and radiographic evaluation of the periodontium with biologic width invasion. BMC oral health 2020;20(1):116.
30. Parma-Benfenali S, Fugazzoto PA, Ruben MP. The effect of restorative margins on the postsurgical development and nature of the periodontium. Part I. Int J Periodontics Restorative Dent 1985;5(6):30–51.
31. Greenberg J, Laster L, Listgarten MA. Transgingival probing as a potential estimator of alveolar bone level. J Periodontol 1976;47(9):514–7.

32. Kan JY, Kim YJ, Rungcharassaeng K, et al. Accuracy of bone sounding in assessing facial osseous-gingival tissue relationship in maxillary anterior teeth. Int J Periodontics Restorative Dent 2017;37(3):371–5.

33. Coslet JG, Vanarsdall R, Weisgold A. Diagnosis and classification of delayed passive eruption of the dentogingival junction in the adult. Alpha Omegan 1977;70(3):24–8.

34. Lee EA. Aesthetic crown lengthening: classification, biologic rationale, and treatment planning considerations. Pract Proced Aesthet Dent 2004;16(10):769–78, quiz 780.

35. Lee EA, Jun SK. Achieving aesthetic excellence through an outcome-based restorative treatment rationale. Pract Periodontics Aesthet Dent 2000;12(7): 641–8, quiz 650.

36. Abou-Arraj RV, Majzoub ZAK, Holmes CM, et al. Healing time for final restorative therapy after surgical crown lengthening procedures: a review of related evidence. Clin Adv Periodontics 2015;5(2):131–9.

37. Listgarten M. Ultrastructure of the dento-gingival junction after gingivectomy. J Periodontal Res 1972;7(2):151–60.

38. Deas DE, Moritz AJ, McDonnell HT, et al. Osseous surgery for crown lengthening: a 6-month clinical study. J Periodontol 2004;75(9):1288–94.

39. Brägger U, Pasquali L, Kornman KS. Remodelling of interdental alveolar bone after periodontal flap procedures assessed by means of computer-assisted densitometric image analysis (CADIA). J Clin Periodontol 1988;15(9):558–64.

40. Pontoriero R, Carnevale G. Surgical crown lengthening: a 12-month clinical wound healing study. J Periodontol 2001;72(7):841–8.

41. Lanning SK, Waldrop TC, Gunsolley JC, et al. Surgical crown lengthening: evaluation of the biological width. J Periodontol 2003;74(4):468–74.

Lip Repositioning Techniques and Modifications

Dimitris N. Tatakis, DDS, PhD, FICD

KEYWORDS

- Esthetics • Dental • Lip surgery • Mouth mucosa surgery • Smiling
- Treatment outcomes • Plastic surgery • Gingiva

KEY POINTS

- Hypermobile upper lip is highly prevalent in patients presenting with excessive gingival display (gummy smile) and represents a common cause of gummy smile.
- Lip repositioning surgery was introduced as an alternative to orthognathic surgery for patients with gummy smile due to hypermobile upper lip.
- Since the original description of the surgical technique, several modifications have been proposed to improve patient experience and stability of clinical outcomes.
- Lip repositioning surgery, a procedure with minimal complications, is effective in significantly reducing gingival display and improving smile esthetics.
- Patients who underwent lip repositioning surgery report high levels of satisfaction with the treatment outcomes and the overall experience.

INTRODUCTION

Gingival display during smile, that is, the exposure of the gingival tissues surrounding the maxillary anterior teeth when smiling, is common. Studies report that 14% to 70% of females[1–6] and 7% to 38% of males present with gingival display,[1–6] that is, they have a high smile. Females are, on average, twice as likely as males to have a high smile, regardless of age or ethnic origin.[1–8] Intrinsically, gingival display is an acceptable component of a pleasing smile; however, smile attractiveness typically decreases when gingival display exceeds 2 to 3 mm, which is termed excessive gingival display.[9–13]

Excessive gingival display, often referred to as gummy smile, is a condition resulting from diverse causes and is often multifactorial. Gummy smile may be due to

This work was supported by the Division of Periodontology, College of Dentistry, The Ohio State University.

Division of Periodontology, College of Dentistry, The Ohio State University, Postle Hall, 305 West 12th Avenue, Columbus, OH 43210-1267, USA

E-mail address: tatakis.1@osu.edu

developmental (eg, due to skeletal development), anatomic (eg, short upper lip), or disease (eg, drug-induced gingival enlargement) conditions, as well as others.[14-17] Among the identified causes of gummy smile, the 2 most common are altered passive eruption,[18-20] usually managed by esthetic crown lengthening,[19,21] and hypermobile upper lip.[14,16]

Hypermobile upper lip has been defined as lip movement, from rest to maximum smile, which exceeds 8 mm.[14] The prevalence of hypermobile upper lip in the population at large is unknown; however, it is highly prevalent in patients with gummy smile. Among North American[22] and Asian[23] adults with gummy smile, more than 85% have hypermobile upper lip. In more than 40% of the cases, it is the sole soft tissue cause identified, and in another 35% to 40% it is combined with altered passive eruption.[22,23] These findings suggest that, for patients with esthetic dissatisfaction because of gummy smile, management of hypermobile upper lip could be an essential approach to provide esthetic improvement and resolution of patient concerns. As with every other therapy, proper diagnostic assessment, patient selection, and thorough treatment planning are essential to obtain optimal results.

MANAGEMENT OF HYPERMOBILE UPPER LIP
Overview of Treatment Approaches

Given the underlying muscular activity and extent of physical translocation that characterize a hypermobile upper lip, most proposed treatment modalities take aim either at curbing the function of the lip-elevating muscles or at placing physical limitations on the tissues' ability to move. Hypermobile lip treatments are categorized into nonsurgical and surgical approaches. A commonly used nonsurgical treatment is application of botulinum toxin.[24-26] When properly applied, botulinum toxin paralyzes specific muscles and results in reduced lip movement during smile.[24-26] This is a transient outcome, lasting 3 to 6 months, and requires repeated application when the toxin effect wears off.[24,26,27]

Surgical treatments for hypermobile upper lip range from procedures that are more invasive, for example, myotomy,[28-30] which severs select muscles implicated in lip lift during smile, to ones that are less invasive, for example, lip repositioning,[31,32] which reduces lip mobility through reduction of the available vestibular mucosa. Myotomy is performed via nasal[29,30] or intraoral[28] access. The reported approaches include: resection of 1 to 2 cm of the levator labii superioris muscle;[28] simple division of the levator labii superioris along with subperiosteal dissection of the alveolar mucosa and gingiva, subcutaneous dissection of the ergotrid area, and maxillary labial frenectomy;[30] and, partial myotomy of the levator labii superioris and insertion of a physical barrier (spacer).[29] Myotomy of the depressor septi nasi muscles, through nasal[33] or oral[34] approach, has been applied in patients with smiles characterized by combination of nasal tip drooping (nasal tip displacing inferiorly and posteriorly), shortened upper lip with a transverse furrow beneath the columella, and with/without excessive gingival display.[33,34] These surgical techniques are effective and result in limited lip elevation during smiling and/or in lip elongation. However, they are nonreversible, due to the transection of the muscles, and may have greater postoperative morbidity.[28]

Lip Repositioning Surgery

Lip repositioning surgery was first described in a 1973 Spanish article by Rubinstein and Kostianovsky,[35] 2 Argentinian plastic surgeons. The original technique described a cosmetic surgery for the "malformation" of the smile, which consisted of the removal of a partial-thickness mucosal strip from the labial aspect of the alveolar mucosa and suture of the apical wound margin to the mucogingival junction (MGJ), thus shortening the vestibule and limiting lip excursion during smile. The described technique included midline frenulum "reconstruction" by creating a fold on the elevated flap. This first report, which introduced lip repositioning as a direct and less invasive alternative to orthognathic surgery, did not provide specific indications or quantitative outcomes. The same authors published the first English-language paper on the technique in 1977.[31] In addition to a detailed description of the surgical procedure, the report stated that lip repositioning was performed on 92 patients with gummy smile, all of whom had improved satisfactorily. However, a "few cases," wherein the excision was "too conservative," experienced recurrence and required a secondary revision procedure. Soon thereafter, in 1979, the technique was described again by Kamer[32] and by Litton and Fournier.[36] The latter report introduced full-thickness elevation and omitted frenulum reconstruction; the investigators added that, in cases of short lip, muscle detachment could be included; they concluded that all their cases had normal appearance after the postoperative edema subsided.[36]

Lip repositioning surgery was introduced to the periodontal and dental cosmetic literature in 2006 and 2007 by Rosenblatt and Simon[37] and Simon and colleagues,[38] who described the original technique, without frenulum reconstruction, and with the coronal incision positioned at the level of the MGJ, instead of 2 to 3 mm coronal to it.[31] Therefore, the surgical technique introduced to the dental community consisted of removal of a single band of mucosa, elevated as a partial-thickness flap, outlined by a coronal incision at the MGJ, an apical incision parallel to the coronal one, and connecting incisions bilaterally, positioned at the level of the projection of the labial commissures during smiling, that is, from the second premolar and up to the level of the second molar, depending on the width of the patient's smile. The apical incision was positioned either at the depth of the vestibule[31] or at a distance that is double the amount of gingival display (in mm) during smile[38,39] but not greater than 10 to 12 mm

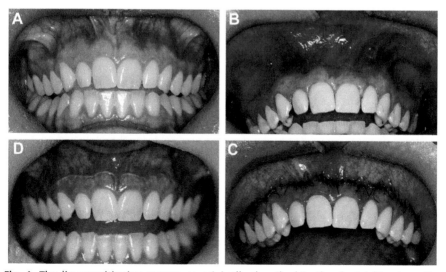

Fig. 1. The lip repositioning surgery as originally described in the dental literature. Retracted views of a case (images presented clockwise): preoperatively (A), following removal of the single mucosal band (B), with sutures in place (C), 6 months postoperatively (D). Note the slight scarring at the level of the mucogingival junction (D).

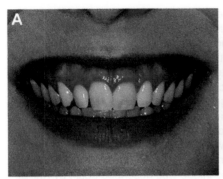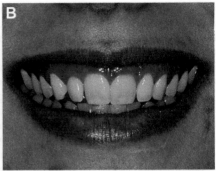

Fig. 2. Preoperative (*A*) and 6-month postoperative (*B*) smile of the same patient treated with the procedure shown in **Fig. 1** (Modified from Andijani RI, Paramitha V, Guo X, et al. Lip repositioning surgery for gummy smile: 6-month clinical and radiographic lip dimensional changes. Clin Oral Investig 2021.). Note the decrease in gingival display and the concomitant increase in vermilion length.

from the coronal incision.[37,38] **Figs. 1** and **2** illustrate a representative case treated with this technique.

The procedure, which is technically reversible, is typically characterized by minor complications. Bleeding during or immediately after removal of the mucosal band is the main intraoperative complication and can be readily managed by application of pressure or electrocautery. Postoperatively, patients usually report mild pain, edema, and tension during smiling or speaking, especially during the first week.[40–42] Rarely, transient numbness[40,42] and paresis,[32] early relapse,[41,43] suture loss,[39,41] ecchymosis,[43,44] mucocele development,[37,38] and formation of double lip[41] have been reported. Healing resulting in slight scarring at the coronal incision line is typically present (see **Fig. 1**).[40] When full-thickness flap elevation and muscle manipulations are incorporated into the procedure (see later), flap dehiscence has been reported,[44] and transient numbness may be more frequent and longer lasting.[44]

The 2 different approaches proposed to determine placement of the apical incision, that is, using depth of the vestibule or twice the amount of gingival display during smile, may or may not result in significant dimensional differences. Novel data from patients with gummy smile indicate that the distance from the central incisor incisal edge to the depth of the vestibule averages 21.2 ± 2.4 mm at rest.[45] When this measurement is considered along with the 10.2 ± 0.9 mm average central incisor length[46] and the 4.4 ± 1.4 mm average gingival width on the same tooth,[47,48] the estimated average apicocoronal distance from MGJ to the depth of the vestibule, at rest, would be 6.5 to 7 mm. Although this distance would appear smaller than the alternative approach (twice the gingival display), this potential difference may be reduced when vestibular depth is determined with the lip (mucosa) stretched. These dimensional considerations are also affected by the coronal incision position. As already mentioned, the proposed coronal incision position has varied; it has been placed 1 mm[49] and 2 mm[50] apical to the MGJ, at the MGJ,[37,38,41,51,52] 1 mm[40,44] and 2–3 mm[31,32] coronal to the MGJ, and 3–4 mm[36] and 4–5 mm[43] apical to the gingival margin. Other investigators have proposed more complex formulas to calculate the apicocoronal dimension of the planned tissue excision, evaluating different landmarks.[50]

Regardless of the choices for placement of the coronal and apical incisions, when contemplating the maximum possible apicocoronal dimension of excised tissue the surgeon should always consider, in addition to the amount of gingival display, the need to (1) maintain a minimum width of 2–3 mm of attached gingiva on all teeth included in the surgical flap design, (2) avoid encroaching on the vermilion border, and, relatedly, (3) allow for postoperative vestibular depth that will not hinder masticatory and other lip functions.

Besides the aforementioned minor variations in basic design, other minor reported modifications include the use of lasers—instead of steel blades—to either mark the location of the incisions or perform the incisions outlining and/or excising the mucosal band area,[42,49,51,53,54] and incorporation of a reversible preoperative outcome assessment trial through temporary use of sutures placed to mimic the end result and thus help patients make informed decisions.[42,53]

Several more distinct modifications have also been introduced. One modification consists of preservation of the midline mucosa (frenulum) and removal of 2 bilateral bands of mucosa (**Fig. 3**) instead of the single mucosal band encompassing the midline.[40,55] This modification was introduced to reduce postoperative morbidity and help maintain the proper position of the labial midline. In contrast, most modifications were introduced to increase postoperative outcome stability and reduce the

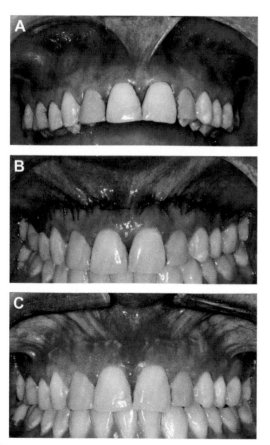

Fig. 3. Modified lip repositioning surgery with retention of the midline maxillary labial frenum. Retracted views of a case: following removal of the bilateral mucosal bands (*A*), with the wounds sutured (*B*), and 6 months postoperatively (*C*). Note the slight scarring at the level of the mucogingival junction (*C*).

occurrence of reported partial relapse.[31,44,52] These modifications include combination of split- and full-thickness flaps,[50] split-thickness flaps combined with periosteal fenestrations,[56] combination of the procedure with botulinum toxin injections,[57,58] use of internal or external anchoring sutures of various designs,[43,50,54,56,58] and integration of muscle management, either through full-thickness[43,44] or partial-thickness[52] flap elevation and blunt dissection of muscle attachments or through application of internal sutures for muscle containment.[59,60]

In cases with subnasal depression, gingival display reduction has been achieved by placement of custom polymethylmethacrylate-based blocks (spacers) after elevation of full-thickness mucoperiosteal flaps, which start at the gingival margin[61,62]; analog[61] and digital[62] approaches have been used for spacer planning and fabrication. Although this approach has been used to achieve repositioning of the lip, it is not directly related to the original lip repositioning procedure.

In cases of asymmetric smile, the technique can be modified to vary the dimensions of the mucosal band removed from each side of the mouth. It can also be applied unilaterally, when indicated.[41,56] Lip repositioning can be used, concurrently or sequentially, in conjunction with other procedures, such as esthetic crown lengthening, when treating patients who present with excessive gingival display of multiple causes.[50,63,64] In such cases, proper treatment planning and procedure sequencing is essential to avoid either unsatisfying esthetic outcomes or the performance of procedures that would be unnecessary.

Clinical and Patient-Reported Outcomes

Despite the numerous earlier reports on lip repositioning surgery, it was not until the 2013 study by Silva and colleagues[40] that quantitative clinical and patient-reported outcomes became available. The study showed that, at 6 months postoperatively, the procedure resulted in approximately 80% reduction of the preoperative gingival display and a concomitant increase in the upper lip vermilion vertical length (see **Fig. 2**; **Figs. 4** and **5**), with a strong correlation between the changes in these 2 clinical parameters.[40] This increase in upper lip vermilion length is considered an esthetic advantage, because vermilion vertical length has been shown to be one of the most significant components of a pleasant smile.[65] Concomitantly, limited gingival display is considered much more esthetically pleasing,[9–13] and gingival display reduction is

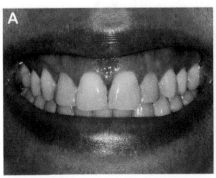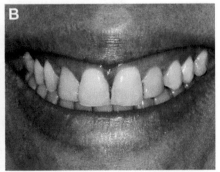

Fig. 4. Modified lip repositioning surgery with retention of the midline maxillary labial frenum. Preoperative (A) and 6-month postoperative (B) smile of the same patient treated with the procedure shown in **Fig. 3**. Note the decrease in gingival display and the concomitant increase in vermilion length.

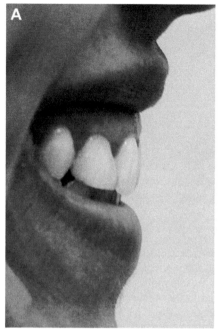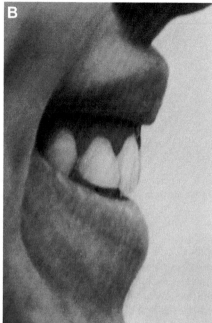

Fig. 5. Profile view of patient shown in **Fig. 4**. Preoperative (*A*) and 6-month postoperative (*B*). Note the changes in gingival display and lip appearance during smile.

a significant determinant of the observed postoperative increase in smile attractiveness of patients with gummy smile, regardless of the procedure involved.[66]

The same 2013 study reported that, at 2.5 years postoperatively, 70% of the patients were very or extremely satisfied with their smile, compared with 0% preoperatively; moreover, 70% thought the amount of postoperative gingival display was about right, when 100% had thought it was too much or way too much preoperatively.[40] Notably, more than 90% of the patients reported that they would be likely to choose to have the procedure again.[40] These first clinical and patient-reported outcomes were subsequently corroborated by several studies that reported similar quantitative outcomes.[49,51,52] It has been recently documented, through clinical and radiographic assessments, that lip repositioning results in significant postoperative reduction of the maxillary vestibular depth, confirming that the procedure works as intended.[45]

Although lip repositioning consistently decreases gingival display and increases vermilion length during smile, recent evidence indicates that it does not cause significant changes to the vertical lip dimensions at rest.[45] Therefore, patients can be reassured that lip repositioning can help improve the esthetics and attractiveness of their smile without affecting their appearance at rest (**Fig. 6**).

Although the procedure is simple and associated with minor complications and high patient satisfaction, partial relapse is a limitation.[31,44,52] Relapse may be noticeable at 12 months or later, and the magnitude apparently depends on surgical technique[40,44,52,54,67,68] and pretreatment conditions, that is, patient selection (Tatakis et al., Unpublished observations).

In 2018, the first systematic review[69] on lip repositioning surgery was published, and, based on the limited available evidence, it was concluded that the procedure resulted in an average 3.4-mm gingival display decrease and, therefore, could be

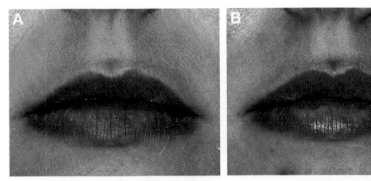

Fig. 6. Frontal view of patient lips at rest (same patient as in **Figs. 1** and **2**). Preoperative (A) and 6-month post-operative (B) images. Note the lack of any lip dimensional changes.

used to treat excessive gingival display. In the last year, several additional systematic reviews have been published.[70–72] The consensus emerging from the systematic reviews is that lip repositioning surgery is effective in reducing gingival display for appropriately selected cases, that incorporation of muscle management approaches might improve long-term outcome stability, and that further research is needed to identify determinants of success and outcome stability.

When dealing with esthetic concerns and procedures aiming to address them, it is important to have independent assessment, excluding the potential bias of the provider or the patient. In the case of lip repositioning surgery, 50 independent raters of varying educational and professional background who evaluated actual pretreatment and posttreatment patient smiles scored the postoperative smiles significantly higher.[66] Similar results were reported when 6 raters assessed preoperative and postoperative patient smiles.[52] These positive independent assessments, in conjunction with the consistently reported high level of patient satisfaction,[40,49,51,52] indicate that the esthetic benefits of lip repositioning surgery can be appreciated by both the patients themselves and those around them.

SUMMARY

Lip repositioning surgery can significantly reduce gingival display caused by hypermobile upper lip and can significantly improve smile attractiveness and patient satisfaction, with minimal complications.

CLINICS CARE POINTS

- Lip repositioning surgery can be used to treat excessive gingival display cases (gummy smile) caused by hypermobile upper lip.
- When additional excessive gingival display causes are present, thorough treatment planning and appropriate procedure sequencing are essential for optimal outcomes.
- Partial relapse can occur and may be minimized by the use of muscle management technique modifications and proper case selection.
- The procedure is effective in reducing gingival display, resulting in high patient satisfaction.

ACKNOWLEDGMENTS

The author is grateful to Drs Reem Andijani, Vanessa Paramitha, and Brian Roy, all former residents at The Ohio State University Advanced Education Program in Periodontics, for their contributions to lip repositioning research projects. The author would also like to thank Dr Andreas Parashis, Dr Shaun Rotenberg, and Ms Laura McCallister for their suggestions and constructive criticism on previous drafts of the article.

DISCLOSURE

The author has nothing to disclose.

REFERENCES

1. Tjan AH, Miller GD, The JG. Some esthetic factors in a smile. J Prosthet Dent 1984;51(1):24–8.
2. Rigsbee OH 3rd, Sperry TP, BeGole EA. The influence of facial animation on smile characteristics. Int J Adult Orthodon Orthognath Surg 1988;3(4):233–9.
3. Peck S, Peck L, Kataja M. Some vertical lineaments of lip position. Am J Orthod Dentofacial Orthop 1992;101(6):519–24.
4. Maulik C, Nanda R. Dynamic smile analysis in young adults. Am J Orthod Dentofacial Orthop 2007;132(3):307–15.
5. Miron H, Calderon S, Allon D. Upper lip changes and gingival exposure on smiling: vertical dimension analysis. Am J Orthod Dentofacial Orthop 2012;141(1): 87–93.
6. Han SH, Lee EH, Cho JH, et al. Evaluation of the relationship between upper incisor exposure and cephalometric variables in Korean young adults. Korean J Orthod 2013;43(5):225–34.
7. Zhang YL, Le D, Hu WJ, et al. Assessment of dynamic smile and gingival contour in young Chinese people. Int Dent J 2015;65(4):182–7.
8. Awad MA, Alghamdi DS, Alghamdi AT. Visible portion of anterior teeth at rest and analysis of different smile characteristics in the Saudi Population of the Jeddah Region. Int J Dent 2020;2020:8859376.
9. Hunt O, Johnston C, Hepper P, et al. The influence of maxillary gingival exposure on dental attractiveness ratings. Eur J Orthod 2002;24(2):199–204.
10. Geron S, Atalia W. Influence of sex on the perception of oral and smile esthetics with different gingival display and incisal plane inclination. Angle Orthod 2005; 75(5):778–84.
11. Kokich VO, Kokich VG, Kiyak HA. Perceptions of dental professionals and laypersons to altered dental esthetics: asymmetric and symmetric situations. Am J Orthod Dentofacial Orthop 2006;130(2):141–51.
12. Ker AJ, Chan R, Fields HW, et al. Esthetics and smile characteristics from the layperson's perspective: a computer-based survey study. J Am Dent Assoc 2008; 139(10):1318–27.
13. Ioi H, Nakata S, Counts AL. Influence of gingival display on smile aesthetics in Japanese. Eur J Orthod 2010;32(6):633–7.
14. Garber DA, Salama MA. The aesthetic smile: diagnosis and treatment. Periodontol 2000 1996;11:18–28.
15. Robbins JW. Differential diagnosis and treatment of excess gingival display. Pract Periodontics Aesthet Dent 1999;11(2):265–72 [quiz: 273].

16. Silberberg N, Goldstein M, Smidt A. Excessive gingival display–etiology, diagnosis, and treatment modalities. Quintessence Int 2009;40(10):809–18.
17. Dym H, Pierre R 2nd. Diagnosis and Treatment Approaches to a "Gummy Smile. Dent Clin North Am 2020;64(2):341–9.
18. Volchansky AC-J. Delayed passive eruption. A predisposing factor to Vincent's infection? J Dental Assoc South Africa 1974;29:291–4.
19. Coslet JG, Vanarsdall R, Weisgold A. Diagnosis and classification of delayed passive eruption of the dentogingival junction in the adult. Alpha Omegan 1977;70(3):24–8.
20. Alpiste-Illueca F. Altered passive eruption (APE): a little-known clinical situation. Med Oral Patol Oral Cir Bucal 2011;16(1):e100–4.
21. Mele M, Felice P, Sharma P, et al. Esthetic treatment of altered passive eruption. Periodontol 2000 2018;77(1):65–83.
22. Andijani RI, Tatakis DN. Hypermobile upper lip is highly prevalent among patients seeking treatment for gummy smile. J Periodontol 2019;90(3):256–62.
23. Çetin MB, Sezgin Y, Akinci S, et al. Evaluating the Impacts of Some Etiologically Relevant Factors on Excessive Gingival Display. Int J Periodontics Restorative Dent 2021;41(3):e73–80.
24. Polo M. Botulinum toxin type A (Botox) for the neuromuscular correction of excessive gingival display on smiling (gummy smile). Am J Orthod Dentofacial Orthop 2008;133(2):195–203.
25. Hwang WS, Hur MS, Hu KS, et al. Surface anatomy of the lip elevator muscles for the treatment of gummy smile using botulinum toxin. Angle Orthod 2009; 79(1):70–7.
26. Sucupira E, Abramovitz A. A simplified method for smile enhancement: botulinum toxin injection for gummy smile. Plast Reconstr Surg 2012;130(3):726–8.
27. Zengiski ACS, Basso IB, Cavalcante-Leao BL, et al. Effect and longevity of botulinum toxin in the treatment of gummy smile: a meta-analysis and meta-regression. Clin Oral Investig 2021;26(1):109–17.
28. Miskinyar SA. A new method for correcting a gummy smile. Plast Reconstr Surg 1983;72(3):397–400.
29. Ellenbogen R, Swara N. The improvement of the gummy smile using the implant spacer technique. Ann Plast Surg 1984;12(1):16–24.
30. Ishida LH, Ishida LC, Ishida J, et al. Myotomy of the levator labii superioris muscle and lip repositioning: a combined approach for the correction of gummy smile. Plast Reconstr Surg 2010;126(3):1014–9.
31. Kostianovsky AS, Rubinstein AM. The "Unpleasant" smile. Aesthet Plast Surg 1977;1(1):161–6.
32. Kamer FM. How I do it"–plastic surgery. Practical suggestions on facial plastic surgery. Smile surgery. Laryngoscope 1979;89(9 Pt 1):1528–32.
33. Cachay-Velasquez H. Rhinoplasty and facial expression. Ann Plast Surg 1992; 28(5):427–33.
34. Benlier E, Top H, Aygit AC. A new approach to smiling deformity: cutting of the superior part of the orbicularis oris. Aesthet Plast Surg 2005;29(5):373–7 [discussion: 378].
35. Rubinstein AM, Kostianovsky AS. Cirugia estetica de la malformacion de la sonrisa. Prensa Med Argentina 1973;60:952.
36. Litton C, Fournier P. Simple surgical correction of the gummy smile. Plast Reconstr Surg 1979;63(3):372–3.
37. Rosenblatt A, Simon Z. Lip repositioning for reduction of excessive gingival display: a clinical report. Int J Periodontics Restorative Dent 2006;26(5):433–7.

38. Simon Z, Rosenblatt A, Dorfman W. Eliminating a gummy smile with surgical lip repositioning. Cosmet Dent 2007;23:100–8.
39. Humayun N, Kolhatkar S, Souiyas J, et al. Mucosal coronally positioned flap for the management of excessive gingival display in the presence of hypermobility of the upper lip and vertical maxillary excess: a case report. J Periodontol 2010;81(12):1858–63.
40. Silva CO, Ribeiro-Junior NV, Campos TV, et al. Excessive gingival display: treatment by a modified lip repositioning technique. J Clin Periodontol 2013;40(3):260–5.
41. Bhola M, Fairbairn PJ, Kolhatkar S, et al. LipStaT: The Lip stabilization technique-indications and guidelines for case selection and classification of excessive gingival display. Int J Periodontics Restorative Dent 2015;35(4):549–59.
42. Gabric Panduric D, Blaskovic M, Brozovic J, et al. Surgical treatment of excessive gingival display using lip repositioning technique and laser gingivectomy as an alternative to orthognathic surgery. J Oral Maxillofac Surg 2014;72(2):404.e1–11.
43. Abdullah WA, Khalil HS, Alhindi MM, et al. Modifying gummy smile: a minimally invasive approach. J Contemp Dent Pract 2014;15(6):821–6.
44. Alammar A, Heshmeh O, Mounajjed R, et al. A comparison between modified and conventional surgical techniques for surgical lip repositioning in the management of the gummy smile. J Esthet Restor Dent 2018;30(6):523–31.
45. Andijani RI, Paramitha V, Guo X, et al. Lip repositioning surgery for gummy smile: 6-month clinical and radiographic lip dimensional changes. Clin Oral Investig 2021;25(10):5907–15.
46. Sterrett JD, Oliver T, Robinson F, et al. Width/length ratios of normal clinical crowns of the maxillary anterior dentition in man. J Clin Periodontol 1999;26(3):153–7.
47. Bowers GM. A Study of the Width of Attached Gingiva. J Periodontol 1963;34(3):201–9.
48. Muller HP, Eger T. Gingival phenotypes in young male adults. J Clin Periodontol 1997;24(1):65–71.
49. Suh JJ, Lee J, Park JC, et al. Lip Repositioning Surgery Using an Er,Cr:YSGG Laser: a case series. Int J Periodontics Restorative Dent 2020;40(3):437–44.
50. Chacon G. Modified lip-repositioning technique for the treatment of gummy smile. Int J Esthet Dent 2020;15(4):474–88.
51. Ozturan S, Ay E, Sagir S. Case series of laser-assisted treatment of excessive gingival display: an alternative treatment. Photomed Laser Surg 2014;32(9):517–23.
52. Tawfik OK, Naiem SN, Tawfik LK, et al. Lip repositioning with or without myotomy: a randomized clinical trial. J Periodontol 2018;89(7):815–23.
53. Jacobs PJ, Jacobs BP. Lip repositioning with reversible trial for the management of excessive gingival display: a case series. Int J Periodontics Restorative Dent 2013;33(2):169–75.
54. Mateo E, Collins JR, Rivera H, et al. New surgical approach for labial stabilization: a long-term follow-up case series. Int J Periodontics Restorative Dent 2021;41(3):405–10.
55. Ribeiro-Junior NV, Campos TV, Rodrigues JG, et al. Treatment of excessive gingival display using a modified lip repositioning technique. Int J Periodontics Restorative Dent 2013;33(3):309–14.
56. Torabi A, Najafi B, Drew HJ, et al. Lip repositioning with vestibular shallowing technique for treatment of excessive gingival display with various etiologies. Int J Periodontics Restorative Dent 2018;38(Suppl):e1–8.

57. Aly LA, Hammouda NI. Botox as an adjunct to lip repositioning for the management of excessive gingival display in the presence of hypermobility of upper lip and vertical maxillary excess. Dent Res J (Isfahan) 2016;13(6):478–83.

58. Vergara-Buenaventura A, Mayta-Tovalino F, Correa A, et al. Predictability in lip repositioning with botulinum toxin for gummy smile treatment: a 3-year follow-up case series. Int J Periodontics Restorative Dent 2020;40(5):703–9.

59. Storrer CL, Valverde FK, Santos FR, et al. Treatment of gummy smile: gingival recontouring with the containment of the elevator muscle of the upper lip and wing of nose. A surgery innovation technique. J Indian Soc Periodontol 2014;18(5): 656–60.

60. Ganesh B, Burnice NKC, Mahendra J, et al. Laser-assisted lip repositioning with smile elevator muscle containment and crown lengthening for gummy smile: a case report. Clin Adv Periodontics 2019;9(3):135–41.

61. Arcuri T, da Costa MFP, Ribeiro IM, et al. Labial repositioning using polymethylmethracylate (PMMA)-based cement for esthetic smile rehabilitation-A case report. Int J Surg Case Rep 2018;49:194–204.

62. Freitas de Andrade P, Meza-Mauricio J, Kern R, et al. Labial repositioning using print manufactured polymethylmethacrylate- (PMMA-) based cement for gummy smile. Case Rep Dent 2021;2021:7607522.

63. Gibson MP, Tatakis DN. Treatment of gummy smile of multifactorial etiology: a case report. Clin Adv Periodontic 2017;7(4):167–73.

64. Sanchez IM, Gaud-Quintana S, Stern JK. Modified lip repositioning with esthetic crown lengthening: a combined approach to treating excessive gingival display. Int J Periodontics Restorative Dent 2017;37(1):e130–4.

65. McNamara L, McNamara JA Jr, Ackerman MB, et al. Hard- and soft-tissue contributions to the esthetics of the posed smile in growing patients seeking orthodontic treatment. Am J Orthod Dentofacial Orthop 2008;133(4):491–9.

66. Silva CO, Rezende RI, Mazuquini AC, et al. Aesthetic crown lengthening and lip repositioning surgery: Pre- and post-operative assessment of smile attractiveness. J Clin Periodontol 2021;48(6):826–33.

67. Dilaver E, Uckan S. Effect of V-Y plasty on lip lengthening and treatment of gummy smile. Int J Oral Maxillofac Surg 2018;47(2):184–7.

68. Foudah MA. Lip repositioning: an alternative to invasive surgery a 4year follow up case report. Saudi Dent J 2019;31(Suppl):S78–84.

69. Tawfik OK, El-Nahass HE, Shipman P, et al. Lip repositioning for the treatment of excess gingival display: a systematic review. J Esthet Restor Dent 2018;30(2): 101–12.

70. Ardakani MT, Moscowchi A, Valian NK, et al. Lip repositioning with or without myotomy: a systematic review. J Korean Assoc Oral Maxillofac Surg 2021; 47(1):3–14.

71. Dos Santos-Pereira SA, Cicareli AJ, Idalgo FA, et al. Effectiveness of lip repositioning surgeries in the treatment of excessive gingival display: a systematic review and meta-analysis. J Esthet Restor Dent 2021;33(3):446–57.

72. Younespour S, Yaghobee S, Aslroosta H, et al. Effectiveness of different modalities of lip repositioning surgery for management of patients complaining of excessive gingival display: a systematic review and meta-analysis. Biomed Res Int 2021;2021:9476013.

Orthognathic Surgery for Management of Gummy Smile

Arash Khojasteh, MS, DMD, PhD[a,b,*], Sadra Mohaghegh, DMD[a]

KEYWORDS

- Gummy smile • Orthognathic surgery • Vertical maxillary excess
- Le Fort osteotomy • Maxillary impaction • Horseshoe osteotomy • Turbinectomy

KEY POINTS

- To measure the amount of impaction, the effect of adjunctive causes (gingival hyperplasia, short lip, hypermobile lip) must be considered.
- For more than 5 to 6 mm of impaction, additional turbinectomy or horseshoe osteotomy has to be considered.
- The possible aging effect of Le Fort 1 osteotomy has to be considered.
- It is recommended to perform surgical intervention after the age of 14 years in girls and 16 years in boys.

INTRODUCTION

Excessive gingival display is defined as the exposure of more than 2 mm of the gingival tissue.[1] Esthetics is the primary goal of treating patients with excessive gingival show.[2] However, proper occlusal harmony and facial proportions can also increase patient satisfaction and quality of life. Considering the cause of the gummy smile, different treatment approaches can be considered to obtain goals.

The excessive gingival show is mainly caused by hypermobility of the upper lip, altered passive eruption, gingival hyperplasia, bony maxillary excess, and other conditions accompanying these issues. Among the mentioned factors, vertical maxillary excess (VME) can be treated with orthognathic surgery in conjunction with orthodontic treatment in some instances.[3,4] Maxillary growth direction is related to genetics, hormone stimulation, and airway conditions. Therefore, considering the cause, improper maxillary growth patterns can be prevented to some extent. For instance, maxillary

---

[a] Department of Oral and Maxillofacial Surgery, School of Dentistry, Shahid Beheshti University of Medical Sciences, Daneshjou Blvd, District 1, Tehran, Tehran Province, Iran; [b] Department of Health and Medical Sciences, University of Antwerp, Antwerp, Belgium
* Corresponding author.
E-mail address: arashkhojasteh@yahoo.com

Dent Clin N Am 66 (2022) 385–398
https://doi.org/10.1016/j.cden.2022.02.003
0011-8532/22/© 2022 Elsevier Inc. All rights reserved.

dental.theclinics.com

vertical hyperplasia can occur due to nasal airway obstruction, which can be prevented by early diagnosis.

VME is classified into 3 categories: total VME leading to posterior and anterior excessive gingival show, posterior VME in which the anterior gingival show is usually normal or reduced, and anterior VME, which usually has dentoalveolar etiology and causes excessive anterior gingival display. Excessive gingival show as a result of total VME is treated with orthognathic surgery. However, anterior VME is treated with anterior segmental impaction or dental intrusion.[5]

The cause of the gummy smile defines the related treatment option. In this article, the main focus is on applying orthognathic surgery for treating patients with the excessive gingival show. Therefore, procedures related to total and anterior VME treatment are discussed. Besides, the alternative treatment options, modifications of commonly performed surgeries, the impact of orthognathic surgery on the soft tissue, complications, and the possibility of posttreatment relapse are also mentioned. In addition, surgical considerations for growing patients with a skeletal gummy smile are provided. Finally, an algorithm representing the surgical treatment options for a skeletal gummy smile is drawn.

DISCUSSION
Clinical Examination

The main aim of the clinical examination is to specify the cause of the gummy smile. Although gingival exposure is used for the primary diagnosis of gummy smile, incisor display is the most reliable factor for surgical treatment planning and differential diagnosis of the etiologic factors. Indeed, higher gingival exposure does not necessarily require a higher maxillary impaction.[1] The vertical profile of the patient cannot be considered in the differential diagnosis. Indeed, gummy smile can be seen in patients suffering from long face syndrome and patients with class 2 deep bite with normal or decreased facial height. Besides, considering that anterior open bite can be related to the dentoalveolar and soft tissue etiologies, it can occur regardless of the presence of VME. In the rest position, a total of 1.5 to 4 mm of the incisors must be displayed.[6] During smiling, the complete tooth show in conjunction with interproximal gingival show occurs. Maximum of 2-mm gingival exposure during smile is acceptable. However, lower amounts are expected in males. During the examinations, it is essential to relax the facial expression muscles. Considering the possibility of lip incompetency in patients with VME, there is a tendency of mentalis muscle contraction for oral competency. Before any surgical procedure, the hypermobility of the upper lip must be analyzed. The upper lip is usually moved about 7 to 8 mm in the full smile. Higher amounts can be considered abnormal function. Besides, having normal tooth show during the rest alongside increased tooth exposure in full smile can be considered as lip hypermobility. However, in patients with combined etiology (eg, VME + hypermobility), the latter approach is not applicable for clinical examination. Any periodontal etiology of the gummy smile has to be detected before surgical treatment planning. Indeed, measuring the transgingival probing depth, clinical crown, and distance from the incisal edge to the cementoenamel junction can help to diagnose gingival hyperplasia, altered passive eruption, or decreased clinical crown due to dental wear (**Fig. 1**). Besides, the patient's medical history must be considered to rule out any gingival enlargement due to systemic conditions or medications. The preoperative length of the upper lip (from the subnasal to the lower border of the upper lip) and the length of the anterior maxilla should be determined to specify whether the excessive gingival show is related to VME or short upper lip.[7] The average lip length

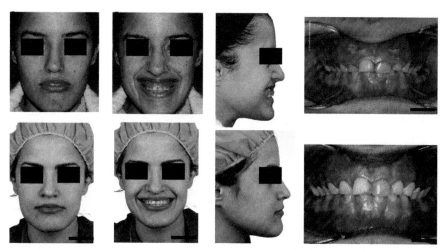

Fig. 1. The excess in the gingival show was because of the gingival hyperplasia and vertical maxillary excess. The patient was treated with 5-mm maxillary impaction and whole arch gingivectomy. Final restorative treatment can enhance the patient's smile line.

is about 20 to 24 mm, which may be more in the younger patients.[8] Patients with short upper lips (<15 mm) may or may not have skeletal problems. Regarding the tooth show, a gummy smile in conjunction with standard or reduced tooth show cannot be related to VME unless in patients with increased length of the upper lip. The possibility of incisor extrusion has to be analyzed. Anterior maxillary overeruption can be seen in conjunction with the disharmonized occlusal plan, deep bite, or tooth wear.[9] Hence, patients with harmonized occlusion are diagnosed with a skeletal gummy smile due to total VME. To sum up, increased tooth show (more than 4 mm), increased lip incompetency (more than 3 mm), and gummy smile are the signs of VME. It must be considered that based on the lip height, amount of VME, and mandibular rotation, lip competency may be seen in patients. Inclination to class II occlusion and mandibular clockwise rotation can also be detected in patients with VME.[10,11] In addition, possible clockwise rotation of the mandible can lower the tongue rest position, leading to deeper and narrower palate vault and posterior crossbite.

Radiographic Analyses

To perform orthognathic surgery for patients with gummy smile, the skeletal etiology (ie, VME) has to be proven. These data can be acquired from lateral cephalometry images. The increased length of the N-ANS line (ie, from nasion to anterior nasal spine with the normal value of 40 mm) indicates the excessive anterior upper facial height. The gummy smile is usually related to the excessive lower facial height, which is defined by ANS-Me line (from the anterior nasal spine to menton with a normal value of 62 mm). Cautions must be taken that increased total anterior facial height, which is analyzed by the Jarabak index and the sum of the abovementioned values, is not necessarily related to the VME. It is essential to assess whether the problem in the Jarabak index is related to the posterior or anterior facial height. Therefore, the Jarabak index should be analyzed considering the anterior facial height as well (**Fig. 2**).

Orthognathic Surgery and Treatment Planning

Garber and Salama[12] divided patients with gingival exposure due to VME into 3 categories: patients with 2 to 4 mm gingival exposure are considered grade 1 and treated

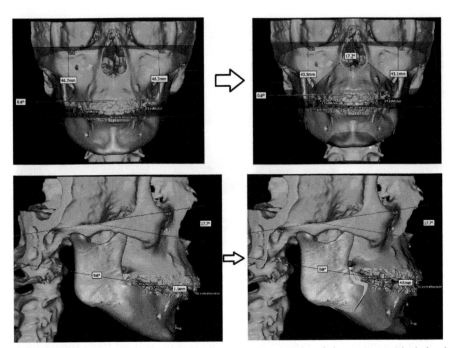

Fig. 2. Changes in the Frankfurt plan and the maxillary height of the patient with skeletal gummy smile.

with orthodontic intrusion, orthodontic and periodontal treatment, or periodontal and restorative treatment. Patients with 4 to 8 mm gingival exposure are considered as grade 2 and are treated with periodontal and restorative procedures or orthognathic surgery. More than 8 mm of gingival exposure is considered grade 3 of VME and is treated by orthognathic surgery with or without periodontal treatment. It must be considered that the values mentioned earlier for gingival display are in patients with normal dentogingival relation, and treatment of gingival hyperplasia and altered passive eruption has to be performed before any classification. The amount of bone removal in the anterior aspect is defined by the upper incisors tooth show. In the posterior portion, the amount of impaction is defined by the position of the mandibular molars following the mandibular autorotation to decrease the possibility of postsurgical posterior open-bite and eliminate the necessity of posttreatment orthodontic treatment. The 3-dimensional position of the upper incisors is the millstone of orthognathic surgery treatment planning. However, Tabrizi and colleagues[13] showed there is about a 20% reduction in the length of the upper lip following the maxillary impaction and the tendency of undercorrection in this surgical procedure exists.[13] The incisor and gingival show are decreased by aging. Therefore, underimpaction may preserve sufficient tooth-gingival show of patients in older ages. In the case of upward-sloped osteotomy and maxillary advancement, the tooth/gingival show will be decreased more than the pure maxillary impaction procedure. The opposite occurs during maxillary advancement with a downward slope.

Le Fort I

Le Fort I (L-1) osteotomies have been considered as the main treatment approach for patients with maxillary vertical overgrowth. Several reference points can be considered for vertical displacement of the maxilla. Steinmann pin and Kirschner wire placed in the nasion can be considered as the reference point. A skin scribe, a suture, or tape can also be used to define the reference point. However, skin movements can decrease the accuracy of the measurements. Besides, considering the complicated 3-dimensional movement of the maxilla following L-1 osteotomy, extraoral landmarks can provide more precise analyses compared with intraoral ones.[14] During the severe VME, 2 osteotomy cuts have to be created to remove a sufficient amount of bone.[15] Besides, it is recommended to avoid removing more than 5 mm of bone in a single L-1 surgery. Further impaction can be obtained by horseshoe osteotomy. However, a modification of L-1 osteotomy has been reported for higher removals. Anehosur and colleagues[16] created the inferior osteotomy cut below the piriform apparatus and closer to the root apexes. The osteotomy included the anterior nasal spine. A V-shaped incision was created to preserve the attachments of the perirhinal muscles and avoid alar base widening. About 8 mm of impaction was achieved using the mentioned modification.

The necessity of adjunctive mandibular surgery has to be defined during treatment planning. Discrepancies less than 3 mm do not require adjunctive mandibular surgery and can be solved by sagittal maxillary movement. Mandibular autorotation can eliminate the necessity of secondary surgery. It has been shown that patients with anterior open bite and a low occlusal plane angle are more prone to have improper postsurgical mandibular rotation.[17] Based on the posttreatment facial profile of the patient, the vertical and sagittal repositioning of the chin has to be performed (**Figs. 3** and **4**). It has been shown that every 1-mm impaction of the maxilla leads to 0.59 mm vertical movement of the chin. In addition, the chin will also move about 0.22 mm in the anterior-posterior direction.[18] In patients with VME accompanied with altered passive eruption, the relation between the gingival margin and cementoenamel junction (CEJ) has to be optimized in the first step and the surgical treatment plan has to be made to reach the tooth show of 2 mm at the rest position.[12] Further removal of the periodontal structures can be performed after the orthognathic surgery based on the patient's demand.[12] In the case of more than 6 to 7 mm of maxillary impaction, it is recommended to perform partial turbinectomy enabling the passive impaction of the maxilla. The intended portion of the turbinate is grasped using a hemostat and removed with dean scissors.[19] Complete turbinectomy is rarely indicated due to the tendency of significant postsurgical complications. Care must be taken to avoid injury of the nasolacrimal duct during turbinectomy.[19]

Horseshoe Osteotomy

Although acceptable results were obtained in patients with a gummy smile after L-1 surgery, severe levels of VME cannot be treated with the L-1 technique alone. Extra impaction of the maxilla requires the trimming of the bone surrounding descending palatine artery. Besides, it has a significant adverse effect on the nasal airway function and the esthetic width of the alar bases of the nose. Considering the possible complications, the horseshoe technique was introduced by Bell and McBride[20] for maxillary impaction of 5 to 15 mm.[21] Indeed, horseshoe osteotomy is performed to impact the dentoalveolar complex and preserve the horizontal palatal segment at a position providing sufficient space for air transmission. Besides, in the case of preexisting nasal airway dysfunctions, it is required to perform horseshoe rather than L-1 osteotomy. Horseshoe osteotomy is made on the superior surface of the down-fractured maxilla. Osteotomy cuts are created from the maxillary sinus and anterior nasal floor to the oral cavity. Caution must be taken to avoid root damage during the osteotomy. Subsequently, the down-fractured maxilla is separated into 2 segments: the

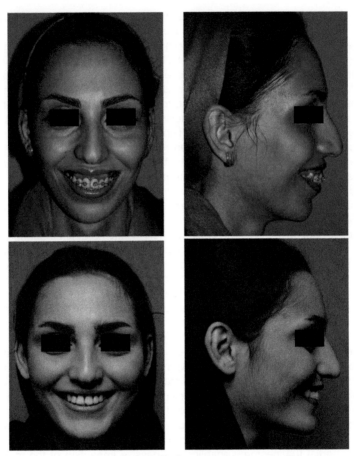

Fig. 3. Superior repositioning of the maxilla (5 mm), with the mandible's counterclockwise rotation (CCWR) and advancement genioplasty. Note that proper soft tissue management can reduce the aging effect of impaction. CCWR can normalize the facial lower third ratio when compared with the middle third in Class II patients.

dentoalveolar complex and palatal components. Although a single horseshoe cut can separate the palatal segment from the dentoalveolar complex, further impaction is not possible in some instances due to heavy traction between the separated bones. Therefore, additional pair of osteotomies can be made to divide the separated palate into 3 segments, increasing the amount of impaction.[22]

Anterior Maxillary Osteotomy

Although patients diagnosed with incisor overeruption are usually treated with orthodontic intrusion, considering the possibility of root resorption and a maximum dental orthodontic intrusion of 10 mm, anterior maxillary osteotomies are considered for severe cases, specifically in adults. Besides, anterior maxillary osteotomy has a shorter treatment duration than orthodontic intrusion.[23] Isolated anterior osteotomy has been widely used for surgical correction of maxillary deformities. However, considering the midfacial harmony acquired through L-1 surgery and its acceptable safety, anterior osteotomies are replaced by L-1 osteotomy.[24] The main indication of anterior

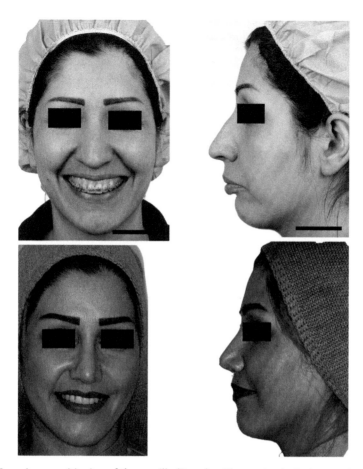

Fig. 4. Superior repositioning of the maxilla (5 mm), with counterclockwise rotation (CCWR) of the mandible and advancement genioplasty in a Cl II deep bite patient. Note the correction of gummy smile and lip incompetency.

dentoalveolar osteotomy is for an anterior open bite. However, in the case of pure anterior VME, the anterior osteotomy method is applicable. Wunderer, Wassmund and Cupar introduced 3 main variations of maxillary anterior osteotomy.[25] All 3 variations enable the anterior-posterior repositioning of the separated maxillary segment. However, the Cupar method is chosen for vertical impaction because it provides direct access to the nasal floor and inferior piriform rim. Besides, it must be considered that only limited levels of impaction can be performed through anterior maxillary osteotomy.[24] It is highly recommended to apply this method in vertical repositioning procedures only when a proper molar relationship presents and the main goal is to decrease the overjet conjunction with excessive gingival show.[25]

COMPLICATIONS
Le Fort 1

Nasal septum deviation is one of the possible complications following L-1 osteotomy, mainly due to insufficient septum resection.[26] Although it has been assumed that the maxillary impaction may cause breathing difficulties, it has been shown that L-1 surgery has no significant impact on velopharyngeal, oropharyngeal, and nasopharyngeal volume.[27] Besides, measurements performed on the amount of nasal airflow showed that impacting the maxilla to some extent can improve the nasal airflow, whereas higher amounts of impaction increase nasal resistance.[28] In the case of pure impaction, there is a significant correlation between the amount of superior repositioning and reduction of the nasal airway volume and increase of the nasal cavity width.[29,30] However, in patients who underwent both impaction and advancement, no correlation was reported.[29] In the horseshoe osteotomy, preserving the soft tissue covered the segmented palatal bone is crucial to avoid postsurgical necrosis. Anterior palatine vessel damage, root damage, and temporarily abnormal palatal shape are the possible complications of additional horseshoe osteotomy.

Stability

At the early postsurgical phase, the fixation plates play the leading role in structural stability. However, following the surgical border ossification, stability is mainly affected by the muscular balance. Indeed, patients with VME usually show weakened masseter and temporalis musculature function, which can be the actual cause of excessive growth.[31] Following the L-1 maxillary impaction, the masseter and temporalis muscles showed significantly improved function during chewing and clenching. However, it was not detected till the firth month postoperatively.[31] It has been shown that maxillary impaction has the least relapse compared with maxillary advancement and inferior repositioning (**Fig. 5**). Indeed, the counterclockwise rotation of the mandible following superior maxillary repositioning provides the proper physiologic support for the maxilla, which increases the stability significantly.[32] Venkategowda and colleagues[33] reported no significant maxillary vertical relapse (ie, 0.5–1.2 mm) 1 year after the L-1 surgery. However, significant dental relapse has been reported. Besides, only 20% of the patients had 2 to 4 mm relapse 5 years after isolated maxillary impaction. Facial

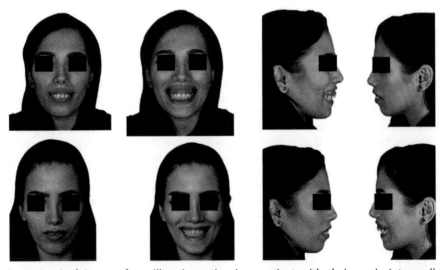

Fig. 5. Total of 9 mm of maxillary impaction in a patient with thalassemia intermedia concomitant with mandibular BSSO surgery. Applying rigid fixation showed proper stability 3 years following surgery.

growth pattern, not technical problems in fixation or the surgical procedure, is the main reason for the postsurgical relapse. It must be considered that the maxillary relapse is regardless of performing mandibular orthognathic surgery.[34]

Soft Tissue Changes

There is no significant difference between the early (ie, 12 months) and late changes (ie, 60 months) of the soft tissue after maxillary impaction.[35] No significant changes in the nasolabial and columella lobular angles can be seen.[36] However, alar base widening and elevation and widening of the nasal tip may occur considering the amount of maxillary impaction and presurgical morphology of the soft tissue.[37] It has been shown that there is no significant correlation between the amount of maxillary impaction and septal deviation, which is mainly due to sufficient septal trimming in the surgeries.[30] However, nasal cavity height significantly decreases following the maxillary impaction. Besides, higher impaction leads to higher amounts of nasal cavity width.[30] Eyelid-brow area is also affected after maxillary impaction (**Figs. 6** and **7**). Carboni and colleagues[38] showed a significantly higher position of the eyelid-brow complex with a more oval eye shape in patients with long face who underwent maxillary impaction. Considering the incision and suturing technique, upper lip thinning and shortening can be expected. Maxillary impaction will also decrease the anterior facial height due to mandibular rotation.

Alternative Approaches

Some compensatory options can be considered for treating skeletal gummy smile. Application of lip repositioning rather than orthognathic surgery in patients with VME has been reported previously.[39–41] Modifications such as detachment of the elevator muscle in cases of a short upper lip,[42] myectomies or partial resection of 1 or 2 levator labii superior muscles,[43] and implantation of an alloplastic or autogenous spacer[44] have been implemented to decrease the possibility of relapse. However, posttreatment relapse still exists. Restricting the superior movement of the upper lip is another treatment option. Several studies reported injection of botulinum with or without conjunctive periodontal surgeries in patients with VME who refused to undergo orthognathic surgery.[45] However, it must be considered that this approach

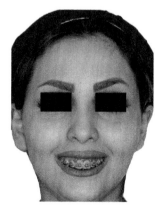 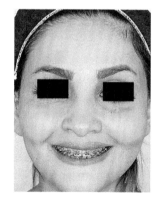

Fig. 6. Soft tissue changes following superior repositioning of the maxilla. Although the gummy smile has been treated, nasal alar widening and the lower lid-eye complex changes showed the aging effect on the patient's frontal appearance (2 years after surgery).

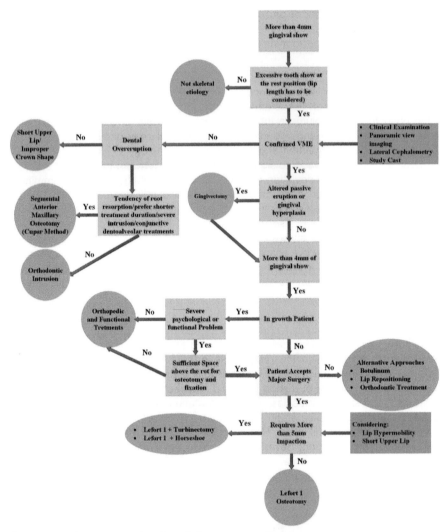

Fig. 7. Surgical treatment planning of the gummy smile.

does not have predictable long-term results, and it is a compromising treatment method for skeletal gummy smiles. Rajagopal and colleagues[46] showed that in patients with less than 5 mm gingival exposure, injecting botulinum can provide about 3.5 mm gingival coverage, which lasts for 7 months. After the second injection, 3 mm gingival coverage can be obtained.[46] However, it will relapse to the preinjection state as well. Botulinum type A is injected into the levator and circumoral muscles, including levator labii superior, levator labii superior alaeque nasi, depressor septi nasi, zygomaticus minor, and orbicularis orris.[47,48] The location of the injection is related to the type of the gummy smile (ie, anterior, posterior, mixed, and asymmetrical). Pregnancy, lactation, allergy to botulinum toxin, lactose and albumin, myasthenia gravis and Charcot disease, and usage of aminoglycoside antibiotic, which improves the action of toxin, are the main contraindications of botulinum injection.[49]

Growing Patients

VME in growing patients can be treated using orthopedic and functional orthodontic appliances (**Fig. 7**). However, there are contradictions in the literature regarding the early surgical management of growing patients with severe skeletal deformities. However, it must be considered that the unesthetic dentofacial appearance of these patients can significantly impact their psychosocial life. There are limited data regarding the proper timing of performing different maxillary surgeries in growing patients. Wolford and colleagues[50] mentioned that the most predictable results are achieved when the surgery is performed after 14 years for girls and 16 years for boys. In the earlier ages, after the orthognathic surgery, although the maxillary vertical overgrowth is not as significant as the presurgical step, there is still the possibility of vertical hyperplasia. Besides, the presence of developing permanent teeth in the alveolar bone complicates the osteotomy procedure. Damage to the roots of the unerupted permanent teeth can cause ankylosis leading to localized alveolar bone defects. It is recommended to postpone the surgical treatment of the growing patient to increase the predictability of the results. However, in the case of severe functional and psychosocial problems, surgery can be performed in the early ages if adequate space for osteotomy and fixation is provided above the developing permanent teeth.[50] To sum up, the following surgical treatment planning diagram is recommended.

SUMMARY

Orthognathic surgery is the optimal treatment option for patients with VME. L-1 osteotomy is the chosen surgical approach for maxillary impaction. However, it can be accompanied by further procedures such as horseshoe osteotomy or partial turbinectomy, usually performed for severe superior maxillary repositioning. It must be considered that the surgical approach is only applicable in patients with total VME and moderate and severe anterior VME. Clinically significant complications such as hemorrhage or major nerve damages rarely happen. Besides, insignificant amounts of relapse have been reported.

CLINICS CARE POINTS

- Turbinectomy or horseshoe osteotomy is applicable for more than 6 to 7 mm of impaction
- It is recommended to treat growing patients after 14 and 16 years in girls and boy, respectively.
- The possibility of 10% lip repositioning following the L-1 surgery has to be considered.
- L-1 surgery has no significant postsurgical complication and relapse and is considered a safe surgical procedure.

DISCLOSURE

The authors have nothing to disclose.

REFERENCES

1. Tomaz AFG, Marinho LCN, de Aquino Martins ARL, et al. Impact of orthognathic surgery on the treatment of gummy smile: an integrative review. Oral Maxill Surg 2020;24(3):283–8.

2. Mahardawi B, Chaisamut T, Wongsirichat N. Gummy Smile: A Review of Etiology, Manifestations, and Treatment. Siriraj Med J 2019;71(2):168–74.
3. Gowri S, Sankar VS, Venkateswaran S, et al. Treatment of an adult patient with a periodontally compromised skeletal Class II malocclusion. World J Orthod 2009; 10(3):233–42.
4. Moure C, Qassemyar Q, Dunaud O, et al. Skeletal stability and morbidity with self-reinforced P (L/DL) LA resorbable osteosynthesis in bimaxillary orthognathic surgery. J Craniomaxillofac Surg 2012;40(1):55–60.
5. Gill DS, Naini FB. Smile Aesthetics: Specific Considerations in the Orthognathic Patient. Orthognathic Surg 2016;214–20.
6. Silberberg N, Goldstein M, Smidt A. Excessive gingival display–etiology, diagnosis, and treatment modalities. Quintessence Int (Berlin, Germany : 1985) 2009;40(10):809–18.
7. Bendrihem R, Vacher C, Fohlen A, et al. Anatomic basis of Le Fort 1 impaction osteotomy: a radiological study. Surg radiologic Anat 2017;39(11):1209–14.
8. Jorgensen MG, Nowzari H. Aesthetic crown lengthening. Periodontol 2000 2001; 27:45–58.
9. Ahmad I. Anterior dental aesthetics: gingival perspective. Br dental J 2005; 199(4):195–202.
10. Ellis E 3rd. The nature of vertical maxillary deformities: implications for surgical intervention. J Oral Maxill Surg 1985;43(10):756–62.
11. Schendel SA, Eisenfeld J, Bell WH, et al. The long face syndrome: vertical maxillary excess. Am J Orthod 1976;70(4):398–408.
12. Garber DA, Salama MA. The aesthetic smile: diagnosis and treatment. Periodontol 2000 1996;11:18–28.
13. Tabrizi R, Zamiri B, Kazemi H. Correlation of clinical predictions and surgical results in maxillary superior repositioning. J Craniofac Surg 2014;25(3):e220–3.
14. Fonseca RJ, Marciani RD, Turvey TA. Treatment Planning in Orthognaric Surgery. In: Oral and maxillofacial surgery3, 3rd. St Louis, MO: Elsevier; 2009. p. 13–30.
15. Posnick J. Sequencing of orthognathic procedures: step-by-step approach. Orthognathic surgery: principles and practice. St Louis, MO: Elsevier; 2014. p. 441–74.
16. Anehosur V, Joshi A, Nathani J, et al. Modification of LeFort I osteotomy for severe maxillary vertical excess asymmetry. Br J Oral Maxillofacial Surg 2019;57(4): 374–7.
17. Peleg O, Mijiritsky E, Manor Y, et al. Predictability of Mandibular Autorotation After Le Fort I Maxillary Impaction in Case of Vertical Maxillary Excess. J Craniofac Surg 2019;30(4):1102–4.
18. Jayakumar J, Jayakumar N, John B, et al. Quantitative Prediction of Change in Chin Position in Le Fort I Impaction. J Maxill Oral Surg 2020;19(3):438–42.
19. Dabir A, Vahanwala J. Orthognathic surgery for the maxilla-LeFort I and anterior maxillary osteotomy. Oral and Maxillofacial surgery for the Clinician. Springer; 2021. p. 1513–48.
20. Bell WH, McBride KL. Correction of the long face syndrome by Le Fort I osteotomy. A report on some new technical modifications and treatment results. Oral Surg Oral Med Oral Pathol 1977;44(4):493–520.
21. Lanigan DT, Hey JH, West RA. Aseptic necrosis following maxillary osteotomies: report of 36 cases. J Oral Maxill Surg 1990;48(2):142–56.
22. Yoshioka I, Khanal A, Kodama M, et al. Postoperative skeletal stability and accuracy of a new combined Le Fort I and horseshoe osteotomy for superior repositioning of the maxilla. Int J Oral Maxill Surg 2009;38(12):1250–5.

23. Hwang BY, Choi BJ, Lee BS, et al. Comparison between anterior segmental os-teotomy versus conventional orthodontic treatment in root resorption: a radiographic study using cone-beam computed tomography. Maxillofacial Plast Reconstr Surg 2017;39(1):34.

24. Bastidas JA. Surgical Correction of the "Gummy Smile". Oral Maxillofacial Surg Clin 2021;33(2):197–209.

25. Gunaseelan R, Anantanarayanan P, Veerabahu M, et al. Intraoperative and perioperative complications in anterior maxillary osteotomy: a retrospective evaluation of 103 patients. J Oral Maxill Surg 2009;67(6):1269–73.

26. Baeg SW, Hong YP, Cho DH, et al. Evaluation of Sinonasal Change After Lefort I Osteotomy Using Cone Beam Computed Tomography Images. J Craniofac Surg 2018;29(1):e34–41.

27. Vijayakumar Jain S, Muthusekhar MR, Baig MF, et al. Evaluation of Three-Dimensional Changes in Pharyngeal Airway Following Isolated Lefort One Osteotomy for the Correction of Vertical Maxillary Excess: A Prospective Study. J Maxill Oral Surg 2019;18(1):139–46.

28. Kim HS, Son JH, Chung JH, et al. Nasal airway function after Le Fort I osteotomy with maxillary impaction: A prospective study using the Nasal Obstruction Symptom Evaluation scale. Arch Plast Surg 2021;48(1):61–8.

29. Ha YC, Han SJ. A 3-Dimensional Analysis of Nasal Cavity Volume After Maxillary Le Fort I Osteotomy. J Oral Maxill Surg 2018;76(6):1344, e1341.

30. Atakan A, Ozcirpici AA, Pamukcu H, et al. Does Le Fort I osteotomy have an influence on nasal cavity and septum deviation? Niger J Clin Pract 2020;23(2):240–5.

31. Priyadarsini P, Muthushekar MR. Longitudinal changes in muscle activity of masseter and anterior temporalis before and after Lefort I osteotomies, An EMG study. Ann Maxillofac Surg 2011;1(2):131–5.

32. Proffit WR, Phillips C, Turvey TA. Stability following superior repositioning of the maxilla by LeFort I osteotomy. Am J Orthod dentofacial orthopedics 1987;92(2):151–61.

33. Venkategowda PR, Prakash AT, Roy ET, et al. Stability of Vertical, Horizontal and Angular Parameters Following Superior Repositioning of Maxilla by Le Fort I Osteotomy: A Cephalometric Study. J Clin Diagn Res : JCDR 2017;11(1):Zc10–4.

34. Jackson TH, Golden BA. Stability of orthognathic surgery. Orthognathic Surg 2016;1:361–72. https://doi.org/10.1002/9781119004370.ch18.

35. Sarver DM, Weissman SM. Long-term soft tissue response to LeFort I maxillary superior repositioning. Angle orthodontist 1991;61(4):267–76.

36. Aydil B, Özer N, Marşan G. Facial soft tissue changes after maxillary impaction and mandibular advancement in high angle class II cases. Int J Med Sci 2012;9(4):316–21.

37. Gill DS, Naini FB, Koudstaal M. The Soft Tissue Effects of Orthognathic Surgery. Orthognathic Surg 2016;341–6.

38. Carboni A, Amodeo G, Perugini M, et al. Morphological Eyelids Changing After Orthognathic Surgery in Long-Face Syndrome. J Craniofac Surg 2019;30(8):e784–7.

39. Dym H, Pierre R 2nd. Diagnosis and Treatment Approaches to a "Gummy Smile. Dental Clin North Am 2020;64(2):341–9.

40. Gabrić Pandurić D, Blašković M, Brozović J, et al. Surgical Treatment of Excessive Gingival Display Using Lip Repositioning Technique and Laser Gingivectomy as an Alternative to Orthognathic Surgery. J Oral Maxillofacial Surg 2014;72(2):404, e401.

41. Deepthi K, Yadalam U, Ranjan R, et al. Lip repositioning, an alternative treatment of gummy smile – A case report. J Oral Biol Craniofac Res 2018;8(3):231–3.
42. Litton C, Fournier P. Simple Surgical Correction of the Gummy Smile. Plast Reconstr Surg 1979;63(3).
43. Miskinyar SAC. A New Method for Correcting a Gummy Smile. Plast Reconstr Surg 1983;72(3).
44. Ellenbogen R, Swara N. The Improvement of the Gummy Smile Using the Implant Spacer Technique. Ann Plast Surg 1984;12(1).
45. Mostafa D. A successful management of sever gummy smile using gingivectomy and botulinum toxin injection: A case report. Int J Surg Case Rep 2018;42: 169–74.
46. Rajagopal A, Goyal M, Shukla S, et al. To evaluate the effect and longevity of Botulinum toxin type A (Botox®) in the management of gummy smile - A longitudinal study upto 4 years follow-up. J Oral Biol Craniofac Res 2021;11(2):219–24.
47. Pedron IG, Mangano A. Gummy Smile Correction Using Botulinum Toxin With Respective Gingival Surgery. J Dent (Shiraz) 2018;19(3):248–52.
48. Naini FB, Witherow H, Gill DS. Surgical Correction of Vertical Maxillary Excess (VME). Orthognathic Surg 2016;448–62.
49. Jaspers GW, Pijpe J, Jansma J. The use of botulinum toxin type A in cosmetic facial procedures. Int J Oral Maxill Surg 2011;40(2):127–33.
50. Wolford LM, Karras SC, Mehra P. Considerations for orthognathic surgery during growth, part 2: maxillary deformities. Am J Orthod dentofacial orthopedics 2001; 119(2):102–5.

Laser-Assisted Gingivectomy to Treat Gummy Smile

Saverio Capodiferro, DMD[a],*, Rada Kazakova, DMD, PhD[b]

KEYWORDS

- Gummy smile • Laser gingivectomy • Laser crown lengthening
- Altered passive eruption • Excessive gingival display

KEY POINTS

- Gingivectomy for a gummy smile correction is a procedure often performed in everyday clinical practice because of the growing popularity of the "smile makeover" procedures. It aims at exposing a greater gingival-incisal length of the clinical crown, often before prosthetic restorations.
- Laser gingivectomy is a safe and mini-invasive alternative to the classic surgical methods—scalpel, piezo surgery, electrocautery, and so forth.
- The advantages of laser surgery are less to no anesthesia, faster, predictable, and uneventful gingival healing, no need for suturing, as well as the possibility to work on patients on anticoagulant and antiaggregant therapy, affected by disease-related disorders of blood coagulation, diabetics, and so forth.
- Lasers can alter the mucosa and gingival tissues without causing bleeding, which enables the clinician also to perform hard tissue crown lengthening by "flapless" remodeling of the bone.

INTRODUCTION

Excessive gingival display (EGD), often referred to as a "gummy smile" or a "high smile line," is the extensive exposure of the gingiva during a smile. It is a common concern among patients, which may compromise the esthetic outcome of the dental treatment. The dentist needs to be familiar with the etiology of the EGD to perform a thorough examination in order to reach to the accurate diagnosis. It is crucial for the adequate treatment of the issue.

[a] Department of Interdisciplinary Medicine, University of Bari "Aldo Moro", Piazza G. Cesare 11, 70100 Bari, Italy; [b] Department of Prosthetic Dentistry, Faculty of Dental Medicine, Medical University – Plovdiv, 3 'Hristo Botev' Boulevard, Bulgaria
* Corresponding author.
E-mail address: capodiferro.saverio@gmail.com

Dent Clin N Am 66 (2022) 399–417
https://doi.org/10.1016/j.cden.2022.02.004
0011-8532/22/© 2022 Elsevier Inc. All rights reserved.

The gummy smile is a nonpathological condition, causing esthetic disharmony in which more than 3 to 4 mm of gingival tissue is exposed when smiling.[1] The anatomic landmarks that have to be in harmony are the maxilla, lips, gingival architecture, and teeth.[1][2] The possible causes can be short lip length, hypermobile lip/hyperactive lip activity, short clinical crown, dentoalveolar extrusion, altered passive eruption (APE), vertical maxillary excess (VME), or gingival hyperplasia.[1][2] The cause is often multifactorial. The accurate diagnosis is essential for the adequate treatment plan and is based on a few consecutive assessments. Patient's medical history gives information about the age and overall health. Facial cephalometric analysis evaluates the facial thirds and can denote VME in cases with skeletal class II relationships. Lip analysis may indicate a short lip, hypermobility of the lip, or both. Dentoalveolar analysis specifies the horizontal and vertical dimension of the clinical crown; a differential diagnosis is made between a short clinical crown due to incisal edge wear and APE. The diagnosis is confirmed by analyzing the incisal edge and the patient's age and determining whether the discrepancy is located at the incisal margin or the gingival margin. Periodontal analysis includes periodontal probing depth, clinical attachment level, presence or absence of gingival recession, which indicates whether the short clinical crown is due to inflammation, gingival hyperplasia or APE. APE is defined as a condition in which the relationship between teeth, alveolar bone, and the soft tissues create an EGD.[2][3] If the cemento-enamel junction (CEJ) can be detected in the gingival sulcus and all other causes have been ruled out, a diagnosis of APE can be made.[2] Determining the etiologic factor(s) is crucial for determining the appropriate treatment options. In cases of short lip or mild VME, lip-repositioning orthognathic surgery is usually required. Hypermobile lip is treated with botulinum toxin A injections, and severe VME can be corrected by orthognathic surgery. Gingival hyperplasia is treated by performing gingivectomy, and APE can be corrected by soft and/or hard tissue crown lengthening.[2][4]

LASER BASICS

The term "laser" (L.A.S.E.R.) is an acronym for "Light Amplification by Stimulated Emission of Radiation". Depending on the optical properties of the tissues, light can interact with them in four different ways: *reflection*, *absorption*, *transmission*, and *scattering*.[5] The main laser–tissue interaction is *photothermic*, which means that laser energy is transformed into heat. The three main photothermic laser-tissue interactions are as follows: 1. *Incision/excision*, 2. *Ablation/evaporation*, and 3. *Hemostasis/coagulation.* Laser-emitting modes play a key role in increasing tissue temperature. The important principle of each mode is that laser energy affects the tissue for a certain period of time, causing thermal interaction. If the laser is used in a *pulsed mode*, the target tissue will have time for cooling before the next pulse. In a *continuous-wave mode*, the operator has to seize the laser action manually to obtain thermal rest of the tissue. Thin or delicate tissue has to be treated in a pulsed mode, so that the amount and speed of the tissue removal is less, but the chances of irreversible thermal damage to the target and adjacent tissue are minimal. Longer pulse intervals also help to avoid heat transfer to the surrounding tissue. Besides, light air cooling or airflow from the surgical aspiration will help cool the tissue. Similarly, when using hard-tissue lasers, water cooling will help prevent microfractures of the crystal structure and will reduce the likelihood of tissue charring. Thick and fibrous tissue, on the contrary, will need more energy to remove it. For the same reason, dental enamel, with its higher mineral content, requires more ablation power than soft carious tissue. In both cases, however, the use of too much heat energy will lead to a delay in recovery and an increase in postoperative discomfort.[5]

Lasers have a wide range of pulse parameters. To allow the tissue to cool, some lasers let the operator change the working time of the impulse, called *pulse width*.

Duty cycle, or also called *emission cycle*, is the time during which the laser is turned on and off. A 10% duty cycle means that the laser is on 10% of the time and is off the remaining 90% of the time. Thin, fragile tissues should be treated with short duty cycles, whereas thick tissues can be treated with longer cycles or continuous-wave mode.[5]

Different laser wavelengths are absorbed in varying degrees, mainly by water, pigments, blood, and minerals.[6] Therefore, laser energy can be reflected, absorbed, transmitted, or scattered, depending on the target tissue composition. The primary absorbents of the specific laser light are called *chromophores*.[5] Water, which is present in all biologic tissues, absorbs maximally the two erbium wavelengths, followed by the two CO_2 wavelengths. On the contrary, water allows passing of more shortwave lasers (eg, diode or Neodymium:YAG [Nd:YAG]). Tooth enamel consists mainly of hydroxyapatite and water. The apatite crystal absorbs the wavelengths of the CO_2 laser and interacts to a lesser extent with the erbium wavelengths. It does not interact with shorter wavelengths. Hemoglobin and the other blood components and pigments, such as melanin, absorb diode and Nd:YAG wavelengths to varying degrees.

Human dental tissues consist of a combination of ingredients, so that the clinician can choose the best laser for each treatment. For soft tissue treatment, it is possible to choose each one of the existing lasers because all the wavelengths are absorbed by one or another component of the soft tissues. For hard tissues treatment, erbium and 9.3 μm CO_2 lasers with very short pulse durations easily evaporate layers of calcified tissue with minimal thermal effect. Short-wave lasers (eg, diode or Nd:YAG) are essentially nonreactive to healthy tooth enamel. Therefore, reconstructing of gingival tissue near the tooth goes smoothly with these wavelengths. Conversely, if soft tissue enters a carious lesion, the erbium laser can remove the lesion and the soft tissue very efficiently, as long as the correct settings for each tissue are applied.[5]

Laser energy is bactericidal, which results in a sterile cut. Moreover, compared with other surgical means, postsurgical bacteriemia is greatly reduced and the healing process is accelerated due to the sealing of blood and lymph vessels.[7] A thorough understanding of laser physics is essential for a predictable outcome.[8]

SURGICAL LASER WAVELENGTHS

CO_2 *laser* wavelengths are 10,600 and 9300 nm and are emitted through an articulating arm or waveguide that ends with a handpiece. Most manufacturers of such lasers offer handpieces with different angles (straight and contra-angle), and different focal points to perform procedures such as evaporation, coagulation, or tissue modification.

Oral soft tissues contain 90% to 97% water. CO_2 lasers' wavelengths are strongly absorbed by water, similar to the erbium ones. Therefore, CO_2 lasers are highly efficient on soft tissues. Soft tissue excision and incision are performed at 100°C, at which intracellular and extracellular water evaporation causes ablation of the biologic tissue.[5] Considering the spot dimension, the reduced mobility of the handpiece and the focus distance, CO_2 laser use on small gingival margins for smile correction may result in irregular gingival profiles.

Erbium lasers currently present with two wavelengths—Erbium:YAG (Er:YAG) at 2940 nm and Erbium,Chromium:YSGG (Er,Cr:YSGG) at 2780 nm. Erbium laser wavelengths are transmitted through semiflexible hollow waveguides, low-OH⁻ fiberoptic cables, or articulated arms. All of them terminate in a handpiece that may use sapphire, quartz, or a hollow metal tip to transfer the energy to the target tissue.[5] These

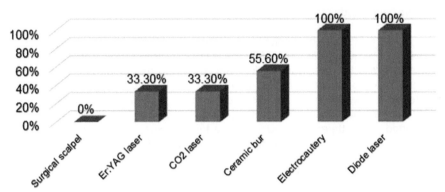

Fig. 1. Influence of the types of surgical instruments on the presence of gingival tissue rupture. *From*: Kazakova RT, Tomov GT, Kissov CK, Vlahova AP, Zlatev SC, Bachurska SY. Histological Gingival Assessment after Conventional and Laser Gingivectomy. Folia Med (Plovdiv). 2018 Dec 1;60(4):610-616. doi:10.2478/folmed-2018-0028. Reproduced with permission of Folia Medica.

wavelengths are strongly absorbed by the water molecules in both soft and hard tissues. Erbium lasers cut soft tissue but with reduced hemostatic ability compared with other soft tissue lasers.[9] With the new technology, providing longer pulse duration and different wavelength configuration, the hemostatic ability has improved.

Erbium and CO_2 lasers with a wavelength of 9300 nm are safe for evaporation of damaged dental tissue. Patients may not even need traditional injection anesthesia, but this requirement is influenced more by the patient's perception of the dental treatment than by the procedure itself. Laser cavity preparation is less traumatic to the pulp tissues than the techniques that involve traditional rotary instruments. Vibration and heat, generated by the rotary instruments, which are the main reasons for the discomfort during the procedures, are less pronounced with erbium lasers.

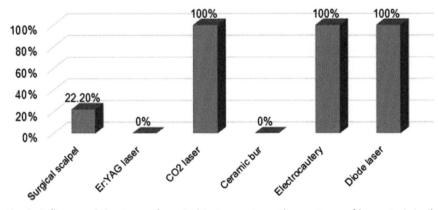

Fig. 2. Influence of the types of surgical instruments on the presence of hemostasis in the depth of the gingival tissue. *From*: Kazakova RT, Tomov GT, Kissov CK, Vlahova AP, Zlatev SC, Bachurska SY. Histological Gingival Assessment after Conventional and Laser Gingivectomy. Folia Med (Plovdiv). 2018 Dec 1;60(4):610-616. doi:10.2478/folmed-2018-0028. Reproduced with permission of Folia Medica.

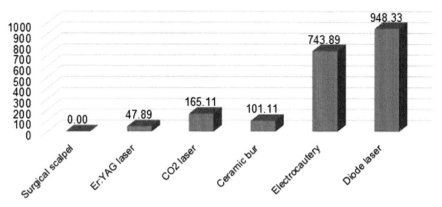

Fig. 3. Coagulation layer width in micrometer depending on the instrument used. *From*: Ka-zakova RT, Tomov GT, Kissov CK, Vlahova AP, Zlatev SC, Bachurska SY. Histological Gingival Assessment after Conventional and Laser Gingivectomy. Folia Med (Plovdiv). 2018 Dec 1;60(4):610-616. doi:10.2478/folmed-2018-0028. Reproduced with permission of Folia Medica.

In order to create higher bond strength, the final preparations have to be etched the conventional way. It is recommended to avoid the techniques that involve smear layer adhesion because lasers remove it. One of the main disadvantages is that lasers with such wavelengths, as well as all the others, are not capable of removing gold or other metal crowns, ceramic, or amalgam restorations.[5] Nevertheless, erbium lasers are generally considered the more suitable devices for soft tissue remodeling in the oral cavity (including gingival tissue) because of their potential for faster healing and atraumatic, predictable, and easily repeatable treatments in esthetic zone.

Diode lasers emit in the wavelength between 810 and 1064 nm, and are compact and portable. They are used for soft tissue procedures and penetrate 2 to 3 mm in-depth, depending on the wavelength and tissue biotype. Wavelengths are absorbed by pigmented structures—*chromophores*, which makes them ideal for cutting mela-notic or highly vascularized soft tissues, as well as for providing hemostasis. Their ef-ficacy can be significantly increased by proper carbonization of the tip. This preparation allows evaporation with a limited peripheral damage of the nonpigmented tissue.[10] Surely, diode lasers are the most widely used in dentistry due to their small dimensions, most affordable cost, as well as for the contextual cut/hemostasis capa-bility, leading to overall advantages especially in gingival cut, vascular lesion nonsur-gical treatment, and oral mucosa lesions removal.[11–19]

Nd:YAG 1064 nm laser wavelengths can be used for numerous soft tissue proced-ures. As with diode and CO_2 lasers, the advantages of Nd:YAG lasers include relatively nonbleeding operative field, minimal edema, reduced surgical time, excellent coagu-lation, and reduced or no postoperative pain.

The main disadvantage of Nd:YAG lasers is the greater depth of penetration into the target tissue. Their wavelengths penetrate deep into the tissue because they are poorly absorbed by water—the main component of the gingiva. The clinician has to be aware of the risk of undesirable collateral tissue damage, of the underlying bone, or of the pulp tissue in particular. Tissue evaporation is slower compared with the other more absorbable wavelengths (eg, CO_2 lasers). The application of a topical photoab-sorbent dye can reduce the absorption time of laser energy. Nd:YAG laser light with any wavelength, directed at the clinical crown or the root, is of particular importance.

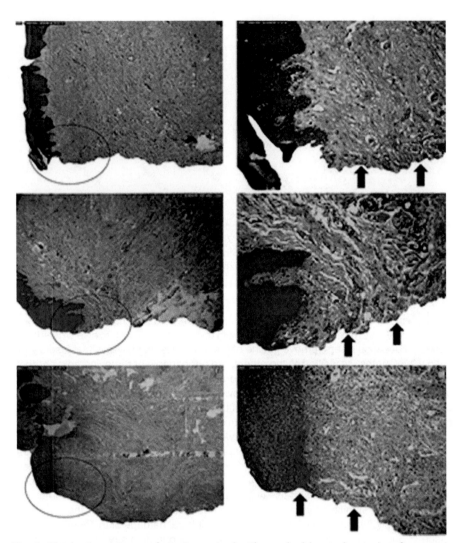

Fig. 4. Histologic specimens of gingiva excised with a scalpel (control group). Left—magnification 40 times, right—magnification 100 times. The arrows indicate the smooth cut surface. There is no rupture, coagulation, and hemostasis in-depth. *From*: Kazakova RT, Tomov GT, Kissov CK, Vlahova AP, Zlatev SC, Bachurska SY. Histological Gingival Assessment after Conventional and Laser Gingivectomy. Folia Med (Plovdiv). 2018 Dec 1;60(4):610-616. doi:10.2478/folmed-2018-0028. Reproduced with permission of Folia Medica.

Pulp heating can be significant and cause inflammation and irreversible damage that can occur if inappropriate operating parameters are used.[20]

GINGIVAL VERSUS COMBINED GINGIVAL AND OSSEOUS SURGERY

After evaluating the cause, arriving at the diagnosis and coming up with a treatment plan that involves raising the gingival margin, it is necessary to determine the extent of the surgery.[8] The choice of the periodontal surgical procedure depends on the gingival architecture, level of crestal bone, gingival biotype, and the amount of

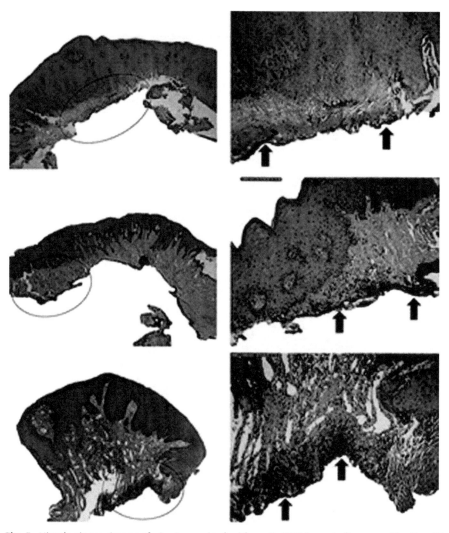

Fig. 5. Histologic specimens of gingiva excised with an Er:YAG laser. Left—magnification 40 times, right—magnification 100 times. The arrows indicate the cut surface. There is rupture in 33.3%, lack of hemostasis in-depth (due to the water cooling) and a very thin coagulation layer (47.9 ± 16.382 μm). (From: Kazakova RT, Tomov GT, Kissov CK, Vlahova AP, Zlatev SC, Bachurska SY. Histological Gingival Assessment after Conventional and Laser Gingivectomy. Folia Med (Plovdiv). 2018 Dec 1;60(4):610-616. https://doi.org/10.2478/folmed-2018-0028.)

keratinized tissue.[21] Crown lengthening is a surgical procedure aiming at revealing a greater gingivo-incisal length of the tooth structure before the prosthetic restoration of the tooth, which involves predictable disclosure of a small amount of gingival tissue alone—*soft tissue crown lengthening*, or both gingival tissue and alveolar bone— *osseous crown lengthening*. Traditional osseous crown lengthening techniques usu- ally include full-thickness flap elevation, ostectomy, and osteoplasty, to determine the new gingival level.[4,22,23]

Soft tissue crown lengthening (gingivectomy) is excision of the gingival margin. Con- ventional methods for performing this procedure include the use of surgical scalpels,

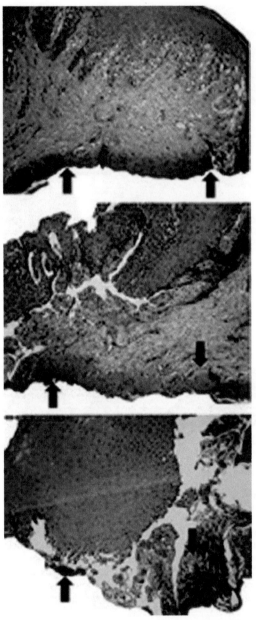

Fig. 6. Histologic specimens of gingiva excised with a ceramic bur. Magnification—100 times. The arrows indicate the cut surface. There is rupture in 55.6%, lack of hemostasis in-depth, and a very thin coagulation layer (101.11 ± 13.176 μm). *From*: Kazakova RT, Tomov GT, Kissov CK, Vlahova AP, Zlatev SC, Bachurska SY. Histological Gingival Assessment after Conventional and Laser Gingivectomy. Folia Med (Plovdiv). 2018 Dec 1;60(4):610-616. doi: 10.2478/folmed-2018-0028. Reproduced with permission of Folia Medica.

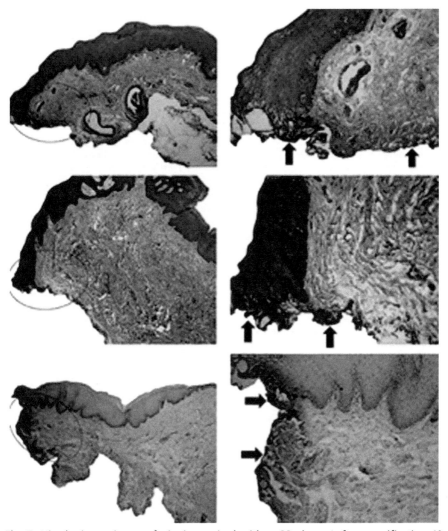

Fig. 7. Histologic specimens of gingiva excised with a CO_2 laser. Left—magnification 40 times, right—magnification 100 times. The arrows indicate the cut surface. There is rupture in 33.3%, presence of hemostasis in-depth, and a thin coagulation layer (165.11 ± 36.440 μm). *From*: Kazakova RT, Tomov GT, Kissov CK, Vlahova AP, Zlatev SC, Bach-urska SY. Histological Gingival Assessment after Conventional and Laser Gingivectomy. Folia Med (Plovdiv). 2018 Dec 1;60(4):610-616. doi:10.2478/folmed-2018-0028. Reproduced with permission of Folia Medica.

periodontal knives, or electrosurgery. In classic gingivectomy, excision is performed apically of the marked bleeding points, but at least 2 mm coronally of the base of the epithelial attachment, to reduce the risk of root surface exposure and biologic width invasion.[8] APE treatment is designated for gingivectomy whenever 3 mm gingival tissue or greater exists from bone to gingival crest, and an adequate zone of attached gingiva will remain after surgery.[21] Gingival hyperplasia, drug-induced or due to hormonal changes, is indicated for soft tissue crown lengthening only.[24,25] Gingivectomy is also indicated for exposure of clear margins for impression taking

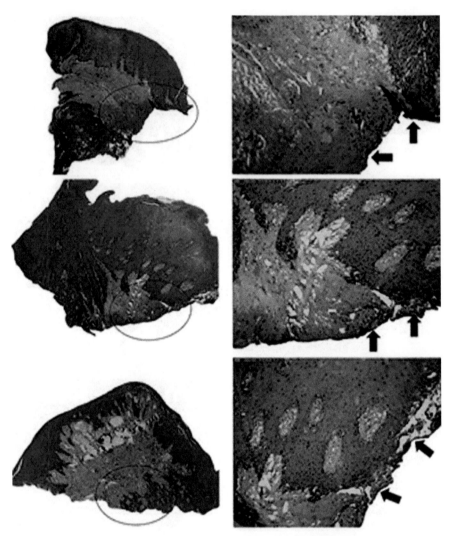

Fig. 8. Histologic specimens of gingiva excised with an electrocautery device. Left—magnification 40 times, right—magnification 100 times. The arrows indicate the cut surface. There is rupture, hemostasis in-depth, and a thick coagulation layer (743.89 ± 69.497 µm). *From:* Kazakova RT, Tomov GT, Kissov CK, Vlahova AP, Zlatev SC, Bachurska SY. Histological Gingival Assessment after Conventional and Laser Gingivectomy. Folia Med (Plovdiv). 2018 Dec 1;60(4):610-616. doi:10.2478/folmed-2018-0028. Reproduced with permission of Folia Medica.

(troughing).[26] Diode, erbium (Er:YAG and Er,Cr:YSGG), and CO_2 lasers are the most commonly used ones for soft tissue remodeling.

Violating the biologic width in patients with "thick and flat periodontal biotype" results in a continuous inflammatory process, and doing so in patients with "thin and scalloped periodontal biotype" results in uncontrolled gingival recession.[8] If raising the free gingival margin to the required esthetic height results in invading the biologic width, then osseous modification is necessary—*bone crown lengthening*.[8] Creating a

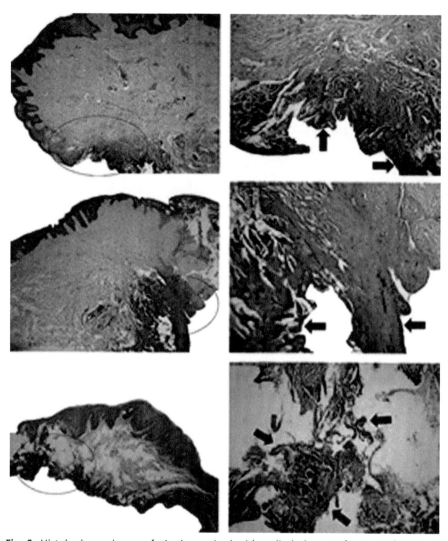

Fig. 9. Histologic specimens of gingiva excised with a diode laser. Left—magnification 40 times, right—magnification 100 times. The arrows indicate the cut surface. There is rupture, hemostasis in-depth, and a thick coagulation layer (948.33 ± 170.990 μm). *From*: Kazakova RT, Tomov GT, Kissov CK, Vlahova AP, Zlatev SC, Bachurska SY. Histological Gingival Assessment after Conventional and Laser Gingivectomy. Folia Med (Plovdiv). 2018 Dec 1;60(4):610-616. doi:10.2478/folmed-2018-0028. Reproduced with permission of Folia Medica.

3 mm distance from the alveolar ridge to the margin of the future restoration results in stable periodontal tissue at that level. The abovementioned distance was proved by Gargiulo and colleagues in 1961 and is based on the biologic width concept.[27] Surgical crown lengthening can be performed after finishing the initial hygienic phase. In APE cases when osseous levels are close to or at the CEJ level, osseous crown lengthening is the adequate treatment solution.[21]

Flap elevation and the following ostectomy and osteoplasty is a traditional method of choice when the crown margin will invade the biologic width. The most commonly

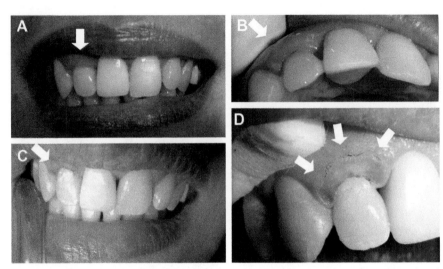

Fig. 10. Alteration of the smile line related to the abundant gingiva of tooth #7 (*A, B*). Gingival remodeling with an Er:YAG laser and its immediate clinical appearance (*C, D*). [From: Capodiferro S, Tempesta A, Limongelli L et al. Minimally invasive (flapless) crown lengthening by erbium:YAG laser in aesthetic zone [version 3; peer review: 2 approved]. F1000Research 2021, 9:1185 (https://doi.org/10.12688/f1000research.26008.3)]

used instruments for this purpose are the rotary ones. Bone recontouring can be achieved conventionally with fissure or diamond burs and water cooling, with bone chisels, or piezoelectric bone surgery.[28,29] This technique reduces irregularities and creates a smooth tissue topography. Sufficient bone is removed in order to create a distance of 3 mm between the bone crest and the finish line of the future restoration. Possible side effects are increased gingival embrasures, root sensitivity, transitional mobility of the teeth and varying degrees of root resorption.[30]

Erbium lasers are more useful in local removal of bone tissue in order to create a new biologic width. By ensuring the careful removal of bone tissues along with the soft tissues in the closed flap technique, the clinician can create a biologic space for the final restoration and often take the impression at the same visit.[5] Erbium lasers have cutting tips handpieces with water cooling, which protect the surgical field from overheating, in contrast to the heat, generated by the rotary instruments' friction. Collateral thermal tissue damage is less with erbium lasers than with conventional techniques.

LASER-ASSISTED FLAPLESS CROWN LENGTHENING WITH BONE RECONTOURING

Because lasers cut with their ends, and not with their sides, a laser may be used in a novel approach to osseous crown lengthening. The so-called "flapless" osseous crown–lengthening procedure can be used to remodel the osseous crest and move it apically. The healing after Er:YAG bone surgery has been reported to be equivalent or faster than that after bur drilling or piezo surgery, and the healing rate observed after "flapless" crown lengthening is equally fast, usually with no evidence of the surgery after 2 weeks.[28,29,31,8] The excellent clinical outcomes in terms of minimal invasiveness, lack of intraoperative and postoperative complications and pain, fast and predictable healing are essentially related to the intrinsic proprieties of the Er:YAG laser light and to the generally recognized gentle laser-oral tissues interaction.[32]

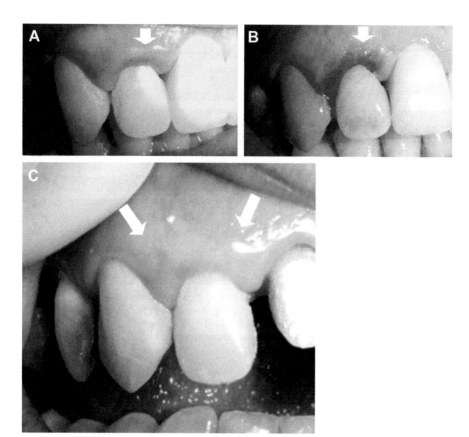

Fig. 11. Second stage after 7 days (*A*). Flapless (through the gingival sulcus) bone recontouring by Er:YAG laser (*B*), and its clinical appearance after 12 days (*C*). (From: Capodiferro S, Tempesta A, Limongelli L et al. Minimally invasive (flapless) crown lengthening by erbium:YAG laser in aesthetic zone [version 3; peer review: 2 approved]. F1000Research 2021, 9:1185 (https://doi.org/10.12688/f1000research.26008.3.)

GINGIVOPLASTY

Soft tissue esthetics' final stage is the design of the gingival tissues surrounding the tooth. The outline of the teeth (especially the anterior sextant) has to be bilaterally symmetric.[8] The gingival trigones (zeniths) are the most gingival points of curvature along the free gingival margins of a tooth. They should be symmetric with the contralateral tooth and in harmony with the adjacent teeth. The position and shape of the interdental papilla must also be considered, especially in cases with diastemata closure. The clinician has to aim at natural appearance and proximal contours that are easy to clean and promote gingival health.[8]

LASER VERSUS CONVENTIONAL GINGIVECTOMY METHODS

In order to explain better the main advantages of laser use in gingival remodeling, it is fundamental to understand what happen to such tissues after laser light interaction. A clinical study conducted by Kazakova in 2017 included histologic specimens from the gingiva of patients aged 18 to 28 years. (*From* Kazakova R, et al. Histologic gingival assessment after conventional and laser gingivectomy. Folia Med 2018;60(4):610 to

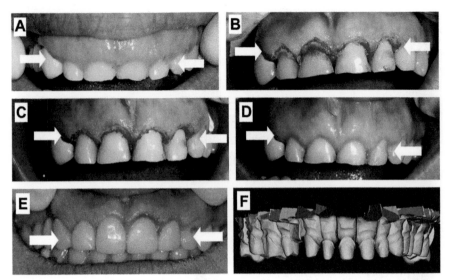

Fig. 12. Severe abrasion of incisors due to bruxism (*A*), Er:YAG laser-assisted gingivectomy (*B*), and contextual flapless bone remodeling (*C*). The clinical appearance after 14 days (*D*), and the following prosthetic rehabilitation (*E, F*). (From: Capodiferro S, Tempesta A, Limongelli L et al. Minimally invasive (flapless) crown lengthening by erbium:YAG laser in aesthetic zone [version 3; peer review: 2 approved]. F1000Research 2021, 9:1185 (https://doi.org/10.12688/f1000research.26008.3.)

6, and Kazakova R. Soft tissue crown lengthening methods. Laser crown lengthening. Lambert Academic Publishing, 2021).[23,33] The samples were excised from patients undergoing soft tissue crown lengthening of the front teeth. One histologic specimen from the gingiva was taken from each patient, and the following surgical instruments were used for the separate surgical excisions:

1. Scalpel (control group)—blade #15c (Hu Friedy, USA).

2. Er:YAG laser—wavelength 2940 nm, Soft Tissue Mode, 50 mJ, 10 Hz (0.50 W altogether) with constant water cooling (LiteTouch, Syneron Dental, Israel).

3. CO_2 laser—wavelength 10,600 nm, in a pulsed mode, with peak pulse power—252 W, duration—200 μs, repetition rate—5 ms, Implant 2nd Surgery mode (DSE, Korea).

4. Ceramic bur—with turbine handpiece (NSK, Ti-Max Z 900 L, 300,000 rpm) without water cooling. (Tissue Trimmer, NTI).

5. Electrocautery device—working mode "Cut" (Kentamed, Bulgaria).

6. Diode laser—wavelength 810 nm, 8 W maximum power a continuous mode with a power of 1.5 W and, depending on the tissue, the power could be increased to 2 W if necessary (FOX, A.R.C. Lasers GmbH, Germany).

The histologic materials, treated with a surgical scalpel in the current study, served as a "control group," and the other 5 surgical instruments—as "test" groups.

After the excisions, the specimens were placed in 10% formalin solution for proper fixation. The biopsies were immersed in paraffin and sections of 5 μm were made. The Olympus CH30 light microscope with 4× and 10× magnifications and the Carl-Zeiss Jena micrometric system Objektmikrometer and Okularmikrometer were used for the pathomorphological study.

Fig. 1 depicts the presence or absence of a microscopic gingival rupture. The scalpel control group demonstrated no rupture. On the contrary, all of the biopsies excised with an electrocautery device and a diode laser were microscopically ruptured. A total of

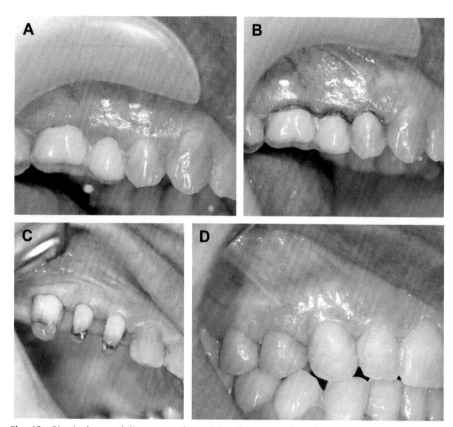

Fig. 13. Gingival remodeling around provisional crowns of teeth #3 and #4, as well as natural tooth #5, performed by diode laser (0.8 W; CW) as no bone recontouring was necessary (*A*). Crowns were exposed, as the smile line needed improvement (*B*). Provisional crowns were remodeled and stayed until to the complete healing, that occurred 8 days later (*C*). The appearance of the final restorations (*D*).

55.6% of the ceramic bur biopsies and 33.3% of the Er:YAG laser and CO_2 laser samples were microscopically ruptured. Hemostasis in-depth was present in all histologic samples excised with a CO_2 laser, electrocautery, and a diode laser. In **Fig. 2**, ceramic bur and Er:YAG laser biopsies showed no hemostasis, whereas it was present in 22.2% in the examined scalpel biopsies. **Fig. 3** demonstrates the width of the coagulation layer in μm. The control samples expectedly showed no coagulation layer (**Fig. 4**). The Er:YAG biopsies had the thinnest coagulation layer—47.9 ± 36.44 μm (**Fig. 5**), followed by the ceramic bur—101.11 ± 13.176 μm (**Fig. 6**) and the CO_2 laser—165.11 ± 36.440 μm (**Fig. 7**). The electrocautery device led to a much wider layer—743.89 ± 69.497 μm (**Fig. 8**), and the widest one belonged to the diode laser samples—948.33 ± 170.990 μm (**Fig. 9-14**). The differences were statistically significant.

CLINICAL CASES PRESENTATION

The following clinical cases are presented to better demonstrate the use of lasers in everyday practice in an outpatient setting.

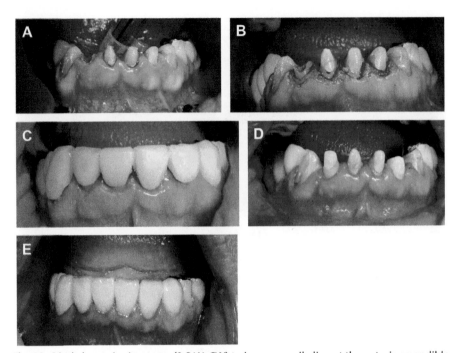

Fig. 14. Diode laser gingivectomy (0.8 W; CW) to improve smile line at the anterior mandible region for prosthetic purposes (*A*). Immediate postoperative appearance (*B*). Healing after 12 days showing good gingival stability (*C, D*). The final prosthetic rehabilitation (*E*). (From: Capodiferro, S. Gengivoplastica con laser a diodo rapidita efficacia mininvasita e predicibilita. Dental Tribune Italy, 2015 Sep 25. Available at: https://it.dental-tribune.com/news/gengivoplastica-con-laser-a-diodo-rapidita-efficacia-mininvasivita-e-predicibilita-2/-.)

DISCUSSION

Traditional scalpel techniques are used to resect tissue in order to provide access and visualization of the target site. Surgical incision with a scalpel may cause loss of gingival attachment with apical repositioning, hyperesthesia, asymmetrical gingival margins after healing due to a more or less unpredictable gingival retraction, as well as postoperative pain and discomfort, typically associated with periodontal surgery. Scalpels do not provide the hemostasis sought when working with highly vascularized tissue.[34] Thus, several other medical devices have been proposed to make the crown lengthening less invasive, including piezo surgery (bone remodeling) and electrocautery device (gingivectomy).[28][29] The use of electrosurgery showed a statistically significant gingival recession, as well as apical migration of the connective epithelium, essentially related to the high working temperature and the associated tissue damage. Deep soft tissue troughing near the bone may result in gingival recession, bone sequestration and necrosis, loss of bone height, involvement of the furcation from the inflammatory process, as well as increased tooth mobility. Electrosurgery is contraindicated around dental implants because of the risk of overheating and should not be used in patients with pacemakers, history of radiation to the jaws, poorly controlled (or uncontrolled) diabetes, blood dyscrasias, immunodeficiency conditions, other diseases that cause a slow healing process.[22] Despite the potential of laser use in dentistry, Christensen reported that soft tissue excision with a surgical scalpel or electrosurgery is faster than the laser excision.[35] This could generally be true, but the creation of a perfect smile is usually not a fast process, as it requires good planning, attention, several clinical evaluations, perfection of previous procedures or modifications, and this as a rule of thumb means more overall time.

Generally, one of the numerous advantages of lasers is that they are safe to use around implants, metal restorations, as well as in patients with diabetes, on anticoagulant or anti-aggregant therapy, and so forth. Laser use leads to minimal or no postoperative pain and can sometimes be selectively applied without anesthesia.[36] Lasers cut the gingival tissues, which results to less bleeding and GR.[37] Laser caused less hemorrhage and inflammation, as well as fast and painless gingival healing. Lasers also present with some other advantages: no or only contact anesthesia is needed; they do not damage hard dental tissues; they are safe to use around metal and metal-ceramic crowns, metal post-and-cores, implants, amalgam fillings; and lasers have a marketing advantage over patients. Faster healing is observed when the wounds made with traditional instruments or lasers are irradiated with Low Level Laser Therapy (LLLT) or Photoactivated Disinfection (PAD) is used.[38]

SUMMARY

Dental lasers demonstrate several advantages for soft tissue dental surgery compared with conventional surgical methods related to their technical characteristics. Due to the excellent coagulation, especially of the surgical lasers, reduced to no need of anesthesia or suturing and faster healing, they demonstrate optimal clinical results. Nevertheless, good knowledge of laser–tissue interaction is required in order to obtain the best predictable results without gingival recession or bone tissue damage.

CLINICS CARE POINTS

- In most cases where a modification of the gingival profile is necessary for aesthetic reasons, lasers simplify the procedures and make them less invasive than conventional surgery and also repeatable when necessary

---

ACKNOWLEDGMENTS

Dr. *S. Capodiferro* would like to thank Prof. Gianfranco Favia (Head of the Dept. of Oral Medicine and Pathology, Faculty of Dental Medicine, Full Professor of the University of Bari "Aldo Moro" — Italy) for the teachings provided over the years; his father Mr. Carmine Capodiferro (Dental Technician), Mr. Daniele De Bellis (Dental Technician), and Mrs. Adelaide Russo (Dental Assistant) for the technical help and collecting cases. Dr. *R. Kazakova* would like to thank her two PhD supervisors: Prof. Angelina Vlahova (Head of Department of Prosthetic Dentistry, Faculty of Dental Medicine, Medical University — Plovdiv, Bulgaria) for her help throughout the years, and Assoc. Prof. Georgi Tomov, DMD, PhD (Head of Department of Periodontology and Oral Diseases, Faculty of Dental Medicine, Medical University — Plovdiv, Bulgaria, and President of the Bulgarian Dental Laser Society) for his support and extensive help with her researches; and to dedicate her work to the loving memory of her dear father — Dr. Torez Kazakov — her inspiration to become a prosthodontist, her teacher, mentor, and biggest supporter through her peaks and valleys.

REFERENCES

1. Pavone AF, Ghassemian M, Verardi S. Gummy smile and short tooth syndrome— Part 1: etiopathogenesis, classification, and diagnostic guidelines. Compend Contin Educ Dent 2016;37(2):102–7.

2. Dym H, Pierre R II. Diagnosis and treatment approaches to a "gummy smile. Dent Clin North Am 2020;64(2):341–9.
3. Chan DK. Predictable treatment for "Gummy Smiles" due to altered passive eruption. Inside Dent 2015;11(7).
4. Verardi S, Ghassemian M, Bazzucchi A, et al. Gummy smile and short tooth syndrome - part 2: periodontal surgical approaches in interdisciplinary treatment. Compend Contin Educ Dent 2016;37(4):247–51.
5. Convissar RA. Principles and practice of laser dentistry. 2nd ed. Elsevier Mosby; 2015.
6. Uzunov T, Uzunova P, Angelov I, et al. Comparative investigation of the penetration of different wavelength visible LED radiation into dental tissue. 15th International School on Quantum Electronics: Laser Physics and Applications 2008;(7027):70271C1-6.
7. Kazakova R. Diode laser gingivectomy healing process. Lambert Academic Publishing; 2021.
8. Magid KS, Strauss RA. Laser use for esthetic soft tissue modification. Dent Clin North Am 2007;51(2):525–45.
9. Tomov G, Bachurska Y, Tashkova D, et al. Pathomorphological distinction between Er:YAG and diode lasers on the excisional biopsy of the oral mucosa. RusOMJ 2013;2(1):0107.
10. Janda P, Sroka R, Mundweil B, et al. Comparison of thermal tissue effects induced by contact application of fiber guided laser systems. Lasers Surg Med 2003;33(2):93–101.
11. Capodiferro S, Loiudice AM, Pilolli G, et al. Diode laser excision of chondroid lipoma of the tongue with microscopic (conventional and confocal laser scanning) analysis. Photomed Laser Surg 2009;27(4):683–7.
12. Capodiferro S, Limongelli L, Tempesta A, et al. Diode laser treatment of venous lake of the lip. Clin Case Rep 2018;6(9):1923–4.
13. Capodiferro S, Maiorano E, Scarpelli F, et al. Fibrolipoma of the lip treated by diode laser surgery: a case report. J Med Case Rep 2008;2:301. https://doi.org/10.1186/1752-1947-2-301.
14. Capodiferro S, Maiorano E, Loiudice AM, et al. Oral laser surgical pathology: a preliminary study on the clinical advantages of diode laser and on the histopathological features of specimens evaluated by conventional and confocal laser scanning microscopy. Minerva Stomatol 2008;57(1–2):1–6, 6-7.
15. Limongelli L, Tempesta A, De Caro A, et al. Diode laser photocoagulation of intraoral and perioral venous malformations after tridimensional staging by high fefinition ultrasonography. Photobiomodul Photomed Laser Surg 2019;37(11): 722–8.
16. Capodiferro S, Tempesta A, Limongelli L, et al. Nonsurgical periodontal treatment by erbium:YAG laser promotes regression of gingival overgrowth in patient taking cyclosporine A: A case report. Photobiomodul Photomed Laser Surg 2019; 37(1):53–6.
17. Capodiferro S, Limongelli L, D'Agostino S, et al. Diode laser management of primary extranasopharyngeal angiofibroma presenting as maxillary epulis: report of a case and literature review. Healthcare (Basel) 2021;9(1):33.
18. Limongelli L, Capodiferro S, Tempesta A, et al. Early tongue carcinomas (clinical stage I and II): echo-guided three-dimensional diode laser mini-invasive surgery with evaluation of histological prognostic parameters. A study of 85 cases with prolonged follow-up. Lasers Med Sci 2020;35(3):751–8.

19. Capodiferro S. Gengivoplastica con laser a diodo rapidita efficacia mininvasita e predicibilita. Dental Tribune Italy. 2015. Available at: https://it.dental-tribune.com/news/gengivoplastica-con-laser-a-diodo-rapidita-efficacia-mininvasivita-e-predicibilita-2/-.

20. Von Fraunhofer JA, Allen DJ. Thermal effects associated with the Nd:YAG dental laser. Angle Orthod 1993;63(4):299–304.

21. Hejazin N, Wehbe C, Wierup M, et al. Diagnosis and treatment modalities of altered passive eruption: Review and a case report of gummy smile. J Case Rep Images Dent 2020;6. 100034Z07NH2020.

22. Carranza NT. Carranza's clinical periodontology. 11th ed. Mosby Elsevier; 2012.

23. Kazakova R. Soft tissue crown lengthening methods. Laser crown lengthening. Lambert Academic Publishing; 2021.

24. Tanev M, Tomov G, Ke JH. Complex management of drug-induced gingival hyperplasia. International magazine of laser dentistry. Int Mag Laser dentistry 2020;1(12):18–21.

25. Yaneva B, Tomov G. Treatment of drug-induced gingival enlargement with Er:YAG laser. Int Mag Laser dentistry 2013;3:34–7.

26. Kazakova R. Gingival retraction methods in fixed prosthodontics. Laser troughing. Lambert Academic Publishing; 2021.

27. Gargiulo AW, Wentz F, Orban B. Dimensions and relations of the dentogingival junction in humans. J Periodontol 1961;32:261–7.

28. Kirpalani T, Dym H. Role of piezo surgery and lasers in the oral surgery office. Dent Clin North Am 2020;64(2):351–63.

29. Lavu V, Arumugam C, Venkatesan N, et al. A present day approach to crown lengthening - piezosurgery. Cureus 2019;11(1):e6241.

30. Maynard JG Jr, Wilson RD. Physiological dimensions of the periodontium significant to restorative dentist. J Periodontol 1979;50:170–7.

31. Lewandrowski KU, Lorente C, Schomacker KT, et al. Use of the Er:YAG laser for improved plating in maxillofacial surgery: comparison of bone healing in laser and drill osteotomies. Lasers Surg Med 1996;19(1):40–5.

32. Capodiferro S, Tempesta A, Limongelli L, et al. Minimally invasive (flapless) crown lengthening by erbium:YAG laser in aesthetic zone. F1000Res 2021;30(9):1185.

33. Kazakova R, Tomov G, Kissov C, et al. Histological gingival assessment after conventional and laser gingivectomy. Folia Med 2018;60(4):610–6.

34. Liboon J, Funkhouser W, Terris DJ. Comparison of mucosal incisions made by scalpel, CO2 laser, electrocautery and constant-voltage electrocautery. Otolaryngol Head Neck Surg 1997;116:379–85.

35. Christensen GJ. Is the current generation of technology facilitating better dentistry? J Am Dent Assoc 2011;142:959–63.

36. Belcheva A, Shindova M. Subjective acceptance of pediatric Patients during cavity preparation with Er:YAG laser and conventional rotary instruments. J IMAB 2014;20(5):631–5.

37. Abdel Gabbar F, Aboulazm SF. Comparative study on gingival retraction using mechanochemical procedure and pulsed Nd-YAG laser irradiation. Egypt Dent J 1996;41:1001–6.

38. Kazakova R. Laser photodynamic therapy and photobiomodulation in prosthodontics. Lambert Academic Publishing; 2021.

Botulinum Toxin and Smile Design

Mario Polo, DMD, MS, FICD[a,b,*]

KEYWORDS

- Gummy smile • Smile esthetics • Excessive gingival display • Asymmetric smiles
- Smile design • Neuromodulators • BOTOX COSMETIC

KEY POINTS

- Smiles with excessive gingival display exceeding 3 mm are considered unattractive.
- Excessive muscular contraction of lip elevator muscles is the etiology in most of these cases.
- Botulinum toxin type A (BTX-A) blocks muscular contraction.
- BTX-A has been proven to be an effective treatment alternative to correct these conditions affecting smile esthetics.

INTRODUCTION

Botulinum toxin type A (BTX-A) was first reported to be used in the face for cosmetic purposes in the early 1990s after being therapeutically used for the treatment of blepharospasm **Table 1**[1] In well-trained hands, injecting this powerful neurotoxin is a simple, effective, and safe procedure. My experience with neuromodulators dates to 2002 when a pilot study using BTX-A for the correction of excessive gingival display (EGD) in subjects with gummy smiles (GS) was performed.[2] On this pioneer evaluation in the use of neuromodulators for the cosmetic improvement of GS, a remarkably beneficial effect was observed and reported. Another clinical trial using a larger sample consisting of 30 subjects with varying degrees of severity in their GS was then conducted: results obtained were quite positive and encouraging, consistently reducing excessive gingival displays to esthetically acceptable levels.[3] The author's clinical experience with OnabotulinumtoxinA for the treatment of GS has primarily been with BOTOX and BOTOX COSMETIC (Allergan, Madison, NJ). All references in this article to BTX-A specifically refer to BOTOX and BOTOX COSMETIC.

[a] Private Practice, Orthodontics and Facial Esthetics, San Juan, PR, USA; [b] Department of Orthodontics, University of Puerto Rico School of Dental Medicine, San Juan, PR, USA
* 702 La Torre De Plaza, 525 F.D. Roosevelt Avenue, San Juan, PR 00918.
E-mail address: drmariopolo@mariopolo.com

Dent Clin N Am 66 (2022) 419–429
https://doi.org/10.1016/j.cden.2022.03.003
0011-8532/22/© 2022 Elsevier Inc. All rights reserved.

dental.theclinics.com

Table 1 Polo's injection protocol for gummy smiles			
Gingival Exposure (mm)	Injection Sites: Number (Location)	Dose (per Side)	Total Units
4.0–5.0	1 (LLSAN/LLS)	2.0 U/side	4.0 U
5.0–7.0	1 (LLSAN/LLS)	2.5 U/side	5.0 U
7.0–8.5	2 (LLSAN/LLS; LLS/Zm)	2.0 U/side	8.0 U
> 8.5	2 (LLSAN/LLS; LLS/Zm)	2.5 U/side	10.0 U

Dose and sites determined according to amount of gingival exposure presented.
  Abbreviations: LLS, levator lavii superioris; LLSAN, levator lavii superioris alaeque nasi; Zm, zygomaticus minor.

BRIEF HISTORY

Produced by the bacterium *Clostridium botulinum*, the initial use of botulinum toxin in medicine was reported in the 1950s by Dr Vernon Brooks, and later in the 1970s, by Dr Alan Scott for the correction of strabismus. It was eventually used for the treatment of blepharospasms, a neuromuscular condition affecting the eyelids, and then used to treat subjects with hemifacial spasms and cervical dystonia.[4] As previously mentioned, the first systematic study of BTX-A in facial rejuvenation was performed in the early 1990s by Jean and Alastair Carruthers, and Botox was then approved for the correction of facial lines in the glabellar region by the US Food and Drug Administration in 2002. This cosmetic effect was attained by means of neuromodulation of the procerus and corrugator supercillii muscles in this facial region. Since then, several other therapeutic and cosmetic applications have been developed and are currently used.

ETIOLOGY OF GUMMY SMILES

Gingival displays of more than 3 mm are considered excessive and unattractive.[5] The etiology of the EGD is multifactorial, and skeletal, periodontal, muscular, and combined factors have been described,[6,7] and treatment should always be determined according to the underlying etiologic factor. When an excessive vertical bony growth of the maxilla is present, a skeletal etiology, the treatment of choice for the correction of the EGD is a Le Fort I osteotomy.[8] When the EGD is secondary to altered passive dental eruption or short clinical crowns, periodontal etiologic factors, gingival reduction by excision (gingivectomy or a surgical crown lengthening) is indicated.[9] Those cases presenting EGD with an underlying muscular etiology and some cases with a combination of etiologic factors that include a muscular component are those in which the use of BTX-A is best indicated. A muscular etiology is present when the upper lip elevator muscles are in a state of hypercontractility when smiling without restriction. At times called lip hypermobility, an excessive elevation of the lip is produced by some of the mimetic muscles responsible to produce a smile.

PREVALENCE

Sexual dimorphism is present in subjects with GS. The prevalence of gingival smiles in female individuals is much higher than in male individuals, with a 96% prevalence in female individuals, as reported by Peck and colleagues.[5]

ANATOMY

Lips are the main facial structures involved in the production of a smile, although other structures, such as the eyes, also interact when conveying a smile, a facial expression of happiness. This happens because the muscles of facial expression are closely inter-leaved one with another, either at their origin or at their insertion. Knowledge of the un-derlying anatomy, as related to the location of muscles, arteries, accompanying veins and nerve endings, their relation to the skin and facial bones, and their actions in pro-ducing facial expressions, is essential when injecting BTX-A. The muscles involved in the production of a smile are the levator labii superioris alaeque nasi (LLSAN), levator labii superioris (LLS), zygomaticus minor (Zm), zygomaticus major (ZM), levator anguli oris (LAO), risorius (R), depressor anguli oris (DAO), depressor labii inferioris (DLI), mentalis (M), depressor septii nasi (DSN), and the orbicularis oris (OO) muscles (**Fig. 1**). It has been previously established that the muscles primarily associated with lip elevation in the production of a smile are the LLSAN, the LLS, the Zm, and the ZM.[10,11]

The LLSAN, LLS, Zm, and the ZM muscles receive their blood supply from the ter-minal branches of the facial artery and the infraorbital branch of the maxillary artery. Blood supply to the LAO comes from various small branches of the labial, infraorbital, and facial arteries, whereas R receives its arterial blood supply via the facial artery and the transverse facial artery at its origin. DAO receives its blood supply from the supe-rior labial branch of the facial artery and the infraorbital branch of the maxillary artery. DLI receives arterial blood supply from the inferior labial branch of the facial artery and the mental branch of the maxillary artery, while the inferior labial branch of the facial artery supplies the M muscle. The DSN is supplied by the superior labial branch of

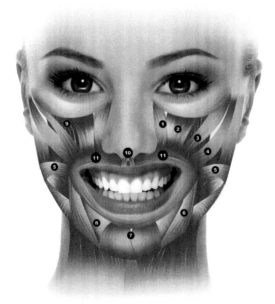

Fig. 1. Facial muscles involved in the production of a smile. 1. LLSAN, 2. LLS, 3. Zm, 4. ZM, 5. R, 6. DAO, 7. M, 8. DLI, 9. LAO, 10. DSN, 11. OO.

the facial artery, whereas the OO has vascular supply mainly from the superior labial and the inferior labial arteries. The nerve supply to all these muscles is provided by the terminal buccal and zygomatic branches of the facial nerve.

PHYSIOLOGY AND MODE OF ACTION

Botulinum neurotoxins are known to have 7 serotypes (A, B, C1, D, E, F, and G). The BTX molecule is a 150-kDa structure composed of a 100-kDa heavy chain, together with a 50-kDa light chain held together by a disulfide bond and an associated zinc metalloprotease. Although the 7 different types of BTX bind at different areas of the nerve membrane and cleave different proteins at the presynaptic nerve terminal, all of them have the same mode of action. All serotypes act by preventing the release of acetylcholine at the neuromuscular junction of striated muscle fibers, thus producing a flaccid paralysis of the muscle.[12]

RECONSTITUTION AND DILUTION

BTX-A is supplied as a vacuum-dried powder in 50-, 100-, and 200-Unit vials that need to be reconstituted with 0.9% normal saline solution without preservatives before being injected. Dilution volumes with saline vary according to the muscle mass to be injected, and the injector's choice of concentration. The BTX-A vial, which is mostly used for cosmetic purposes, is the 100-U vial. The most common dilution protocol used consists of adding 2.5 mL of a 0.9% normal saline solution to a 100-U vial. This dilution will result in a 4.0-U/0.1-mL concentration. For the 50-U vial, using half of these volumes will result in the same concentration, whereas for the 200-U vials, 2x the saline volume will produce the same concentration.[13]

PATIENT EXAMINATION, SELECTION, AND INTERVIEW

The most important factor contributing to a successful treatment outcome, regardless of which, is patient selection. When evaluating a person with a chief complaint of "showing too much gum tissue when smiling," the clinician should first assess the reason why an EGD is present. The etiology needs to be accurately established, for treatment options should be based on the existing etiologic factor because these options should not be used indiscriminately.[14]

The use of BTX-A for GS with a muscular etiology, excessive contraction resulting in extreme upper lip elevation or hypermobility, is the treatment of choice.

Besides an EGD, these subjects also present with a short vertical dimension at the mid-portion of the upper lip at the philtrum, and a thin upper lip vermillion border. In those presenting a "canine smile" type of smile, the gingival exposure extends even more posteriorly, into the premolar and even the molar area.

Quantification of the amount of EGD present is essential because all GS are not the same. EGDs exceeding 4 mm, even up to 15 mm, may be clinically observed. On examination, the clinician should determine and record the amount of EGD present, together with the patient's smile type. Care should be used when considering its use in individuals presenting GS together with a hypotonic or flaccid upper lip. If asymmetry is present, further assessment and planning are essential, and patients should be clearly informed of this and other existing conditions (eg, asymmetric lip elevation, canting of the maxilla, facial asymmetry, mandibular laterognathia). The presence of these and other factors might influence results and interfere with the patient's expectations.

Clinicians should carefully evaluate the patient's expectations regarding this procedure and learn about their degree of satisfaction with results attained with previous cosmetic procedures. Dealing with patients expressing high levels of dissatisfaction with the results of a previous procedure or unrealistic expectations, is a situation that needs to be closely evaluated during this initial session. Thorough written documentation of facial findings and conversation details addressed during the patient's interview must be performed. Photographic documentation, both before and after the injection procedure, is also essential.

DOSE

It is highly advisable to inject varying doses according to the severity of the GS, as learned from the clinical trials initially performed,[2,3] and throughout my clinical experience during the past 20 years successfully injecting BTX-A for GS correction.

During the 2 phases of the first trial, it was established that smaller BTX-A doses of 1.5 U/injection site could not effectively treat subjects with more severe degrees of EGDs. After the second trial, it was observed that higher doses of 2.5 U in subjects with milder degrees of EGD were not as esthetically pleasing as those obtained in more severe cases.

Varying doses according to the severity of the gingival display were then established, and my injection protocol was accordingly modified and clinically used for more than 4 years. This first revision of the initial injection protocol was reported in 2013 in the journal *Plastic Reconstructive Surgery*.[15] In 2016, a second revision with a subtle dose modification was published in the journal *Aesthetic Surgery*.[16] This injection protocol remains the one currently used. It is based on a classification of GS based on the degree of severity and is summarized in the accompanying table (**Table 1**). Pleasing results have been obtained by using these doses. The injection sites remain the same as those originally used with the LLSAN, the LLS, and the Zm muscles being the target muscles. The injection sites for the correction of GS by means of BTX-A injection, the Polo Injection Points,[17] are shown in **Fig. 2**.

INJECTION TECHNIQUE

Upper lip elevator muscles originating in the zygomatic bone present a triangular and inferiorly converging pattern, eventually inserting mostly into the superiorly located fibers of the OO muscle, whereas some of their fibers also insert into the skin of the

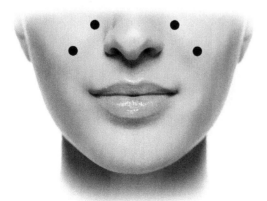

Fig. 2. Polo Injection Points. These points demonstrate the approximate injection location. Exact injection points should be individually determined by means of palpation and animation, as described in the text.

upper lip. The more medially located muscles, the LLSAN, LLS, and Zm pull the upper lip upward (elevation), whereas others more laterally located tend to pull the upper lip laterally and horizontally. These laterally positioned muscles (ZM, LAO, and R) should be avoided to prevent undesired, unesthetic results in the patient's smile. The LLSAN, LLS, and Zm determine the amount of elevation of the upper lip. At their utmost inferior portion near their insertion at the OO, these muscles tend to present proximity, over-lapping, and even interleaving of their fibers. For this reason, these were the target muscles selected for injection during my 2005 preliminary study and continue being so. Because undesired esthetic results could arise by injecting muscles located too far laterally, near the ZM area, the author recommends avoiding such injections.

All in all, in the technique here presented, the target injection sites are the conver-gence area of the LLSAN and the LLS, and the convergence area of the LLS and the ZMi, at the Polo Injection Points[17] (see **Fig. 2**). They are clinically determined on an individual basis for each patient by means of palpation and facial animation and are subject to variation from one individual to another. Factors such as facial dimensions, facial type, and ethnicity, determine this variability, as reported by L.G. Farkas and colleagues.[18] The most superior set of the Polo Injection Points, corresponding to the area where the LLSAN and the LLS approximate each other, is determined by deep digital palpation with the index finger to locate the canine fossa, and further corroborated by muscle animation while still maintaining finger pressure at this area. They usually are located 0.5 cm lateral to the mid-portion of the lateral aspect of the nose. The second set of points, the crossover area of the LLS and the Zm, is located approximately 1.0 cm inferiorly and laterally, and always above the level of the OO muscle, is determined mostly by animation (smil-ing), followed by superficial palpation detecting contraction of these muscles. Again, individualization according to facial type and dimension is critical to attain pleasing esthetic results.

The area is anesthetized with a 5% lidocaine cream for 15 minutes. After removing the anesthetizing cream, the area is thoroughly sanitized with 70% isopropyl alcohol swabs, and the injection preselected points are marked. The use of ice pads before and after injection is recommended because of their additional numbing of the skin and production of localized vasoconstriction, thus reducing discomfort, and reducing the risk of bruising. The BTX-A vial is reconstituted and diluted with a preservative-free 0.9% normal saline solution, as previously explained. The author's dilution choice is 2.5 mL for the 100-U vial, and 1.25 mL for the 50-U vial, both dilutions producing a 4.0 U/0.1 mL injected; 1.0 mL tuberculin syringes with 32G one-half inch needles are used. The desired number of units are then injected at each of these sites. Results attained by this off-label minimally invasive modality for the correction of EGD (GS) are observed within 2 to 5 days postinjection. There is minimal discomfort associated with the procedure and results are highly predictable.

OTHER USES FOR ESTHETIC SMILE ENHANCEMENT

BTX-A has successfully been used by the author for the correction of asymmetric smiles in patients with GS in whom upper lip elevation is greater on one side, as compared with the other side. Also, it has been used in some individuals presenting unilateral upper lip elevation and in persons presenting excessive unilateral lower lip depression secondary to excessive contraction of the DLI muscle.

Careful selection of the injection site(s) and treatment dose is needed when injecting these individuals, and it should be attempted only by experienced injectors because unesthetic results may happen.

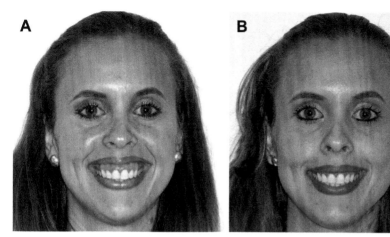

Fig. 3. Full-face smiling photographs of a 30-year-old female patient with a Grade 4 GS of 8.6 mm. (*A*) Before BTX-A injection with 2.5 U/site at 4 sites. (*B*) Two weeks after injection: 8.5-mm reduction in gingival display was attained.

CONTRAINDICATIONS

BTX-A is contraindicated in individuals with hypersensitivity to any botulinum toxin preparation or to any of the components in the formulation. Infection at the injection site is another contraindication. The presence of certain neurologic conditions and other medical conditions may contraindicate treatment with BTX-A. Some prescription and over-the-counter medicines may cause serious side effects. Its use during pregnancy may affect fetus formation. It is unknown if botulinum toxin passes into breast milk during lactation. Adequate evaluation of the medical history is essential before its use.

COMPLICATIONS

Complications arising when using BTX-A usually are site-specific, although there is always the possibility of a distant spread of toxin effect. Some side effects may be serious and even life-threatening. Injectors should familiarize themselves with pertinent medical information provided in the package insert before using BTX-A. When using low doses for the correction of GS, complications are usually few. The most

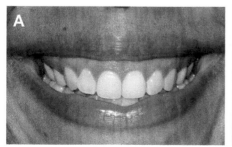
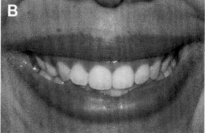

Fig. 4. Close-up smiling photographs of a 32-year-old female patient with a Grade 1 GS of 4.7 mm. (*A*) Before BTX-A injection with 2.0 U/site at 2 sites. (*B*) Two weeks after injection: 3.2-mm reduction in gingival display was attained.

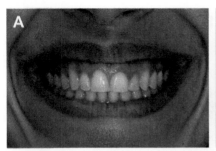
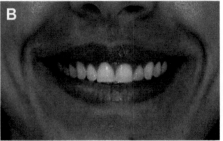

Fig. 5. Close-up smiling photographs of a 37-year-old female patient with a Grade 2 GS of 5.4 mm. (*A*) Before BTX-A injection with 2.5 U/site at 2 sites. (*B*) Two weeks after injection: 5.4-mm reduction in gingival display was attained.

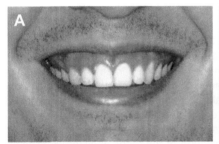
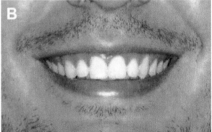

Fig. 6. Close-up smiling photographs of a 30-year-old male patient with a Grade 3 GS of 7.3 mm. (*A*) Before BTX-A injection with 2.0 U/site at 4 sites. (*B*) Two weeks after injection: 6.3-mm reduction in gingival display was attained.

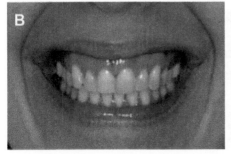
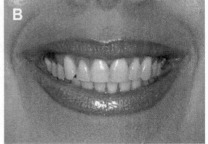

Fig. 7. Close-up smiling photographs of a 31-year-old female patient with a Grade 4 GS of 8.5 mm. (*A*) Before BTX-A injection with 2.5 U/site at 4 sites. (*B*) Two weeks after injection: 8.5-mm reduction in gingival display was attained.

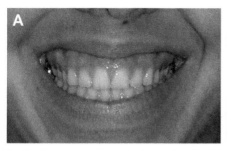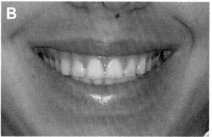

Fig. 8. Close-up smiling photographs of a 21-year-old female patient with an asymmetric bilateral GS, Grade 4 (8.5 mm) right, Grade 3 (7.0 mm) left. (*A*) Before BTX-A injection with 2.5 U/site on the right side and 2.0 U/site on the left side. (*B*) Two weeks after injection: approximately 8.5-mm reduction in gingival display was attained on the right side and 7.0 mm on the left side.

common complications, although infrequently observed, are bruising and tenderness at the injection sites. Smile asymmetry or excessive ptosis or drooping of the upper lip could take place if injection sites are not adequately selected or if dose guidelines are not followed. Injection of BTX-A is a relatively safe procedure when used for the correction of GS with underlying excessive muscle activity. A sound understanding of facial anatomy and adequate training in using neurotoxins is essential.

IMMUNORESISTANCE

For the past 20 years during which I have been injecting BTX-A for the correction of GS, and of thousands of injection sessions for this purpose, only one patient has not had BTX-A correct her EGD condition. This 30-year-old woman had the procedure done on 3 occasions, at a 4-month interval from each other, and using a higher dose on each consecutive session. No change in the upper lip's vertical position was observed in any of these 3 injection sessions. Immunologic resistance to BTX-A is suspected.

CLINICAL CASES

Before and after photographs illustrating the results attained by the author using the technique herein described are enclosed. **Fig. 3** presents before and after full-face photographs of a 30-year-old female patient with canine smile and a severe degree

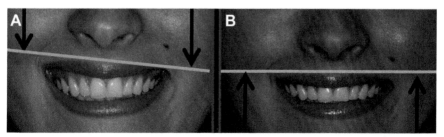

Fig. 9. Close-up smiling photographs of a 22-year-old female patient with an asymmetric unilateral GS on the right side. (*A*) Before BTX-A injection with 1.5 U on the right LLSAN/ LLS site. (*B*) Two weeks after: a significant improvement of the asymmetric smile can be observed.

of gingival display. **Figs. 4–7** present before and after photos of patients with varying degrees of GS. Two patients with asymmetric smiles are presented in **Figs. 8** and **9**: one with a bilateral anterior and posterior GS (see **Fig. 8**), and another patient presenting an asymmetric excessive unilateral anterior GS resulting from excessive contraction of the right-side upper lip elevator muscles (see **Fig. 9**).

CLINICS CARE POINTS

Pearls
- Injection of BTX-A at specific target sites is a minimally invasive treatment alternative for the correction of GS
- This procedure is cost-effective
- Outcomes are effective and predictable

Pitfalls
- Esthetic results could be compromised when incorrectly injected or inadequate doses used
- Results are temporary

DISCLOSURE

Author has nothing to disclose.

REFERENCES

1. Carruthers JD, Carruthers JA. Treatment of glabellar frown lines with C. botulinum-A exotoxin. J Dermatol Surg Oncol 1992;18:17–21.
2. Polo M. Botulinum toxin type A in the treatment of excessive gingival display. Am J Orthod Dentofacial Orthop 2005;127:214–8.
3. Polo M. Botulinum toxin type A (Botox) for the neuromuscular correction of excessive gingival display on smiling (gummy smile). Am J Orthod Dentofacial Orthop 2008;133:195–203.
4. Brin MF, Hallett M, Jankovic J. Preface. In: Brin MF, Hallett M, Jankovic J, editors. Scientific and therapeutic aspects of botulinum toxin. Philadelphia: Lippincott Williams & Wilkins; 2002. v-vi.
5. Peck S, Peck L, Kataja M. The gingival smile line. Angle Orthod 1992;62:91–100.
6. Robbins JW. Differential diagnosis and treatment of excess gingival display. Pract Periodontics Aesthet Dent 1999;11:265–72.
7. Garber DA, Salama MA. The aesthetic smile: diagnosis and treatment. Periodontol 2000 1996;11:18–28.
8. Schendel SA, Eisenfeld J, Bell WH, et al. The long face syndrome: vertical maxillary excess. Am J Orthod 1976;70:398–408.
9. Coslet JG, Vanarsdall R, Weisgold A. Diagnosis and classification of delayed passive eruption of the dentogingival junction in the adult. Alpha Omegan 1977;70:24–8.
10. Rubin LR. The anatomy of a smile: its importance in the treatment of facial paralysis. Plast Reconstr Surg 1974;53:384–7.
11. Pessa JE. Improving the acute nasolabial angle and medial nasolabial fold by levator alae muscle resection. Ann Plast Surg 1992;29:23–30.
12. Singh BR. In: Brin MF, Hallett M, Jankovic J, editors. Scientific and therapeutic aspects of botulinum toxin. Philadelphia: Lippincott Williams & Wilkins; 2002. p. 75–88.
13. BOTOX® COSMETIC [package insert]. Madison, NJ: Allergan; 2021.

14. Polo M. Gummy smile treatment: a 40-year journey. AJO-DO Clinical Companion 2022. https://doi.org/10.1016/j.xaor.2022.01.007 (in press).
15. Polo M. A simplified method for smile enhancement. Plast Reconstr Surg 2013; 131:934e–5e.
16. Polo M. Commentary on: botulinum toxin for the treatment of excessive gingival display: a systematic review. Aesthet Surg J 2016;36:89–92.
17. Polo M. Sorriso Gengival:Visão Ortodôntica – Uso da toxina botulínica. In: Kahn S, Tavares Dias A, editors. Sorriso gengival. Brasil: Quintessence Publishing; 2017. p. 277–302.
18. Farkas LG, Katic MJ, et al. International anthropometric study of facial morphology in various ethnic groups/races. J Craniofac Surg 2005;16(4):615–46.

Lip Augmentation

Shohreh Ghasemi, DDS, Msc[a],*, Zahra Akbari, MD[b]

KEYWORDS

- Lipofilling • Hyaluronic Acid fillers • Facial esthetic • Aging • Fat transfer • Fascia

KEY POINTS

- Smile reconstruction can be revolutionized by filler material for volume augmentation of lips.

INTRODUCTION

The procedure of facial rejuvenation, particularly lip augmentation, has become increasingly popular. To obtain optimal patient outcomes, a thorough understanding of perioral anatomy as well as the structural features that define the aging face is required.

Despite the fact that techniques and technology are constantly evolving, hyaluronic acid (HA) dermal fillers remain to be the most popular esthetic treatment. In some cases, a combination therapy involving neurotoxic and volume restoration produces better results. The best perioral and lip rejuvenation approach has the longest efficacy duration, the lowest complication rate, and the greatest esthetic results.[1]

Angular, radial, and vertical lines of the perioral lines are caused by genetics, intrinsic aging, sun exposure, and repetitive muscle twitching of the orbicularis oris. As a result, patients' needs in the treatment of this anatomic area can range from relatively simple lip enhancement to a holistic treatment with sequential correction of perioral wrinkles. For the regeneration of this area, a variety of materials have been described. Dermal fillers are currently the most popular and widely used lip enhancers, although there is still no consensus on the optimum material for filling soft tissue of the face, particularly the perioral region.[1–3]

Throughout history, several methods have been used to change one's look for spiritual reasons, as well as to comply to esthetic standards. The lips, as a distinguishing feature of the face, offer a one of great opportunity for facial esthetic enhancement. In medicine, there has been a paradigm toward preventative health and a desire to delay or even reverse the aging process. This study highlights perioral anatomy, describes aging of the lower face, and reviews procedures for perioral rejuvenation through volume restoration and muscle control while acknowledging that product technology, skill sets, and cultural ideals are constantly evolving.

[a] OMFS Department, Augusta University, 1120,15 th Street, Augusta, GA 30912, USA; [b] Medical Spa, Tehran, Iran
* Corresponding author.
E-mail address: sghasemi@augusta.edu

Dent Clin N Am 66 (2022) 431–442
https://doi.org/10.1016/j.cden.2022.02.005
0011-8532/22/Published by Elsevier Inc.

Lip Histology

When we observe and magnify the lip laterally by microscope, we have 3 portions histologically. The external portion is the skin lip. The medial portion is the vermilion border of lip (transitional zone), and the inner layer is labial mucosa. The skin area is covered by a thin, stratified squamous keratinized epithelium, the skin extends to the red margin, which forms the red zone of the lips, called transitional zone. As we acknowledged, the epithelium is thinner and covered by a keratinized squamous epithelium but less cornified than the epidermis that lacks hair follicles. The vermilion zone is lined by a thick keratinized, stratified squamous epithelium and hair follicles are lacking. The numerous, densely packed dermal papillae of the lamina propria allow blood vessels close access to the surface, imparting a red color to this zone. The inner surface of the lip is lined by the mucosal epithelium, a thick, moist stratified squamous epithelium; a stratum granulosum is absent. Minor salivary glands (labial glands) are located in the submucosa beneath the lamina propria. The minor salivary glands produce both serous and mucous secretions. Mucosal epithelium also lines the cheeks, floor of the mouth, and the ventral surface of the tongue. The minor salivary glands of the lip, also called labial glands, produce both serous and mucous secretions; their ducts empty into the vestibule of the oral cavity. The epithelium and surface of the inner lip lie above this image. These glands are located in the submucosa near the fibers forming the orbicularis oris muscle (**Fig. 1**).[4]

Perioral Anatomy

The epidermis, subcutaneous tissue, orbicularis oris muscle fibers, and mucosa are the layers of the lips. From the base of the nose to the mucosa inferiorly and to the nasolabial folds laterally, the upper lip extends. The lower lip is curvilinear, extending from the mucosa inferiorly to the mandible and laterally to the oral commissures.

The white roll, a raised patch of pale skin circumferential at the vermilion–cutaneous junction, highlights the vermilion border and considered as an essential landmark during lip augmentation. This elevation of the vermilion connects at a V-shaped dip in the center of the top lip to form the Cupid's bow.[1-4]

The philtral columns, which are generated from decussating fibers of the orbicularis oris muscle, are 2 elevated vertical pillars on the cutaneous upper lip. The philtrum is the ensuing midline depression. During augmentation treatments, these distinguishing features of the top lip should be preserved. The upper and lower lips are supplied by the superior and inferior labial arteries, which are branches of the facial artery. Deep

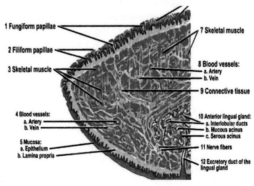

Fig. 1. Lip histology.

injection of the upper lip between the muscle layer and the mucosa can cause harm to the anastomotic arch of the superior labial artery; consequently, caution should be used in this location. Injections into the vermilion and lower lip can be done safely and without fear of vascular damage. The translucency of capillaries in the superficial papillae gives vermilion its red color. The dense sensory nerve network and capillary plexus at the papillae make the lip a highly vascular and sensitive tissue.

The Metric System

Using a specific caliper and the golden ratio as a reference, we devised our technique. As a compliment to Phidias, the sculptor and builder of the Parthenon and many other classical era Greek monuments, the golden ratio, or phi number, is symbolized by the Greek letter. The Phi number is an irrational number of the order 1.618033988 that is obtained when a line a + b is sectioned so that (a + b)/a = 1.618. It was first defined as the golden ratio by the Greek mathematician Euclid in the tenth of his 13 books of *Elements*. Evidence of its occurrence across a wide range of mathematical, biological, and natural systems has been recorded for millennia, based on the belief that it reflects great beauty.[5] It has also occurred in many artistic masterpieces and architectural wonders throughout history, such as Da Vinci's paintings and the Parthenon, and it is, briefly, an attempt to geometrically and mathematically express the enthralling mystery of beauty. We used this number in our method, despite its subjective nature, to identify the right injection spots.[1,5]

Lip Esthetics

A pronounced Cupid's bow, a well-defined vermillion border, upturned corners of the mouth, fullness in the center that fades out toward the mouth, symmetry between the left and right sides, philtrum length of 12 to 15 mm, a thinner upper lip protrusion compared with the larger lower lip, and a balanced upper and lower lip are the basic principles of ideal lips. The golden ratio, which is 1:1.6, is used to calculate the ideal upper lip to lower lip ratio in frontal view. However, lip esthetics alter over time, eras, and races; however, voluptuous lips with enhanced volume are also lovely and appealing.[6] In particular, the current ideal female-lip ratio in White women has just been discovered to be 1:1. To better understand what patients think to be the optimal lip ratio, we performed a survey in 2008 to compare their preferences to expert perspectives and use the results as a guiding tool during the patient–doctor consultation process.

Lip Enhancement and Contour

Definition

- It is essential to avoid product accumulation in any filler injection; hence, a retrograde linear threading approach is always preferred over a big bolus. It is usually done from the medial to the lateral side (5 mm laterally to the commissure), with each hemi-lips being checked for symmetry. We divide the upper lip into thirds and treat the central portion with injections along the philtrum lines through Cupid's bow, according to the no-touch technique.[7,8]

In fact, a simple lip enhancement can be properly treated with blunt cannulas, allowing for less invasiveness and damage when treating a big area. When a finer treatment is required, however, the use of a needle is almost required because it allows for a more uniform injection and helps with refinements and minor asymmetries. HA is a naturally occurring highly hydrophilic glycosaminoglycan polymer that was first isolated more than 70 years ago. Rooster combs, umbilical cord, vitreous fluid, tendons, skin, and bacterial cultures are also common sources for HA purification. An average-sized human is made up of about 15 g of HA, which is largely present in the extracellular matrix of connective tissues and acts as the foundation for the dermis, fascia, and other tissues.

Every day, about a third of the HA in the human body is replaced. The enzyme hyaluronidase easily breaks down the naturally occurring molecule. As a result, chemical modification of these molecules through cross-linking is required to produce an effective filler. Cross-linking increases surface area and thus reduces the surface area available for degradation.[5]

The hydrophilic property of HA is critical to its clinical utility; 1 g of HA can bind 6 L of water. This property enables it to maintain the hydration of the intracellular matrix in which cells are structured, preserving tissue volume and supporting surrounding tissues. HA is also unique in that it has no antigenic specificity because it is not species-specific or tissue-specific. As a result, in clinical use, it has a very low risk of allergic reaction. The purification source and, more crucially, the size of the molecules in the HA products now available varies.[9,10]

This property, in particular, is responsible for each product's distinct characteristics. The "'cement" that holds the collagen "bricks" together has been described as HA products.[7,8]

Methods and Techniques

- Not just for assessing treatment benefits and potential adverse effects but also for medicolegal purposes, well-focused pretreatment images should be taken. Anteroposterior and lateral projections should be used, as well as static and dynamic (smiling and whistling) features, and any asymmetries should be appropriately assessed and addressed. Cleaning with an antibacterial solution is usually recommended.

Lipofilling by Fat Transfer

Alternative to artificial fillers and implants is using your own tissue for lip augmentation. Using your own tissue for lip augmentation is called autologous lip augmentation. Fat transfer is one type of autologous lip augmentation and is another great option for lip augmentation. Similar to lip fillers, fat transfer to the lips is an in-office procedure. Fat transfer to the lips is performed under local anesthesia.

During fat transfer to the lips, fat is harvested from abdomen (around the belly button), purified, and transferred into lips. Fat transfer to the lips takes about 60 to 90 minutes to perform. The patient can go home the day of the procedure. Lips augmented with fat stay plump for 5 years or longer. The complications of lipofilling of fat transfer are minimal and include bruising, swelling, pain, infection, necrosis, and calcification.[11,12]

Tissue Grafting (Fascia Grafting)

There is another type of autologous lip augmentation. In addition to using fat for lip augmentation, a piece of your own skin or dermis can be used for lip augmentation. During this type of autologous lip augmentation, skin is removed from the lower stomach area. Sometimes, a C-section scar can be resected and used for lip augmentation. Sometimes, the skin removed during a facelift can be used for lip augmentation [13].

After the skin is resected, the top layer of the skin (epidermis) is removed. The remaining piece of skin is a strip of dermis and is rolled into a cigar-like shape. This piece of dermis is then inserted into your lips. This type of autologous lip augmentation is also an in-office procedure and can be performed under local anesthesia. The duration of the dermal transfer to lips procedure ranges from 60 to 90 minutes. The patient can go home the day of the procedure. Your lips should retain their shape and volume for 5 years or more.

Limitations

In general, most defects can be repaired, but smaller defects have a better chance of retaining function and form. If the defects are less than 2 to 3 cm, there is a better chance of having enough tissue in the surrounding area to reconstruct. Even when the defects are larger, the surgeon can still use the flaps to do reconstruction. If the defects become very large, the function and form that is acceptable in those situations is different than a smaller defect.

Adverse Effect or Side Effects

Because perfusion of the vessels and blood flow is crucial to the viability of any flap, people who are diabetic or smokers are at a higher risk for complications. Smokers can have a higher risk of complications such as flap necrosis. Fortunately, flaps and surgeries in the facial region are very rich in blood supply; hence, many of these flaps will still be successful. Patients who need any kind of reconstruction should stop smoking. They should also have their blood sugar under control if they are diabetic to lower the chance of getting an infection. Nutrition is important so patients should have adequate nutrition and adequate protein in order to heal their wounds.[11,12]

Injection Technique

- HA is the most often used dermal filler because it is regarded both safe and effective. We used HA with the following qualities in our patients: 3/6 cross-linking, 25 mg/g concentration.[13,14]
- The injection is made into the vermillion through the vermillion border when the goal is to restore volume. To avoid lip vessels, insert a 30-gauge needle at an oblique angle (30°) and no more than 2.5 mm deep at each specified point of the vermillion border. Bend the needle at 2.5 mm to keep the appropriate needle depth measure. Slowly move forward. Small boluses of 0.05 to 0.1 mL of HA are slowly injected at each needle's site, totaling 1 to 1.5 mL in both lips per session. The HA injection is done in a retrograde linear threading technique.
- The injection is done into the vermillion border in order to restore the shape. It is vital to avoid injecting into the white roll at this stage because the hydrophilic HA causes a blunted lip margin, which could be attributable to the area's distinct histologic properties. At a parallel angle, insert a 30-gauge needle at each specified position of the vermillion border. Because this delicate area of the lip is more prone to false outcomes, we strongly advise using only 0.02 to 0.4 mL of HA. Slowly injecting HA in a retrograde linear threading technique is done.
- Depending on the individual's anatomy, assess the lips for any asymmetry and inject 0.05 to 0.1 mL in the desired location if necessary.[9,10]

Normal-volume lips

- Although there is lovely volume (vermillion) and definition (vermillion border), patients are asking for a more projected vision. Injections into the vermillion are used to increase volume and correct any asymmetries. After 15 days, a reassessment is arranged, and if necessary, more volume is added. Each session should only contain 1 to 1.5 mL of HA (**Figs. 2** and **3**).

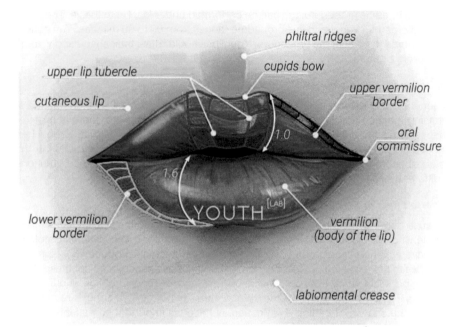

Fig. 2. Lip Anatomy: 8 zones of lip injection by the anatomy.

Thin lips

Patients with genetically acquired atrophic lips choose to have a gorgeous pout instead. The upper lip is commonly deficient in volume, with both lips and the lower lip being less common. The goal is to get the desired result while considering the expansion qualities of soft tissue. To do so, inject 0.5 to 1 mL of HA into the vermillion of the thinner lip in the first session to address the ratio. Inject 0.5 to 1 mL of HA into

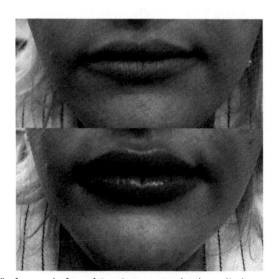

Fig. 3. Lip filler (before and after of 1 syringe, normal volume lips).

both lips as soon as the desired ratio is achieved, usually in the second or even third session.

The sessions are spaced 30 days apart to allow the tissues to adapt to the HA placement and to continue until the desired volume is reached. If there are any asymmetries, we inject additional HA on the proper side of the lip to rectify them. The next stage is to define and shape the lips using the same step-by-step approach, injecting a moderate amount (0.02–0.4 mL) of HA into the vermillion border. After 15 days, reassess and, if necessary, add additional HA to achieve a better definition (**Figs. 4** and **5**).

Aged thin lips

Some aging indications include the absence of the vermillion border, soft tissue volume loss, upper lip lengthening, and vertical lines. These people want to seem younger. We like to correct the volume first by injecting HA into the vermillion, and then the shape by injecting HA into the vermillion border, similar to how we correct the volume in thin lips. Because lips have limited expansion qualities, the usage of 0.5 to 1 mL in each session, every 30 days, is critical. Aged lips, in contrast to thin lips, require less HA (up to 0.5 mL) per session, requiring more sessions to attain the required natural results. HA can also be injected into the upper lip's vertical lines as early as the first session. In terms of the longevity of the outcomes, we have found that after using 3 1 mL syringes, the intended results can endure for a long time, with the average period for a patient to return to our office to maintain the initial result being 12 to 18 months (**Figs. 6** and **7**).

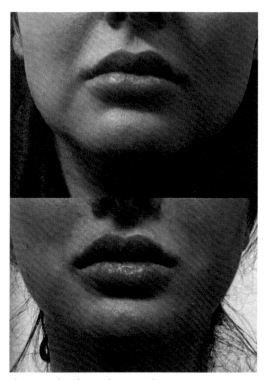

Fig. 4. Normal lip volume and reshape the vermillion zone.

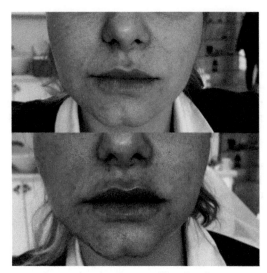

Fig. 5. Thin lip augmentation and make the vermillion border more prominent.

Modern Technique (Latest Technique of 2020)

What is the Russian lip filler technique?

Russian lip fillers are inspired by Russian nesting dolls and their perfectly coiffed lips. The Russians are regarded as one of the most attractive people on the planet. You have probably observed how Russian women present supermodel-like lips without the dreaded "duck pout."

By injecting additional volume and lift into the middle of the lips, the Russian procedure enhances the Cupid's bow to resemble a heart-shape, whereas the sides of the lips stay reasonably in line with the face. The end product is doll-like, yet with a natural fullness and plumpness. Instead of a wider volume, this design emphasizes the center of the lips, giving you the coveted baby-doll aspect. Unlike standard lip fillers, the

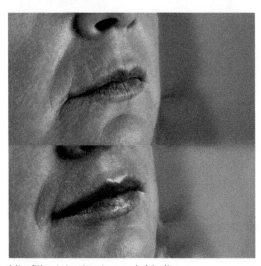

Fig. 6. Conventional lip filler injection in aged thin lip.

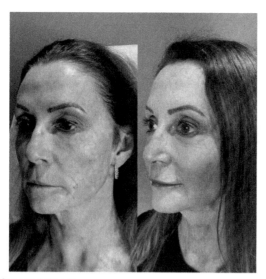

Fig. 7. Lipofilling for aged thin lip.

product is injected vertically, starting at the base of the lip and working outward toward the lips' border. Most standard lip filler procedures focus on restoring volume. The method is more complex with Russian lips.

The therapy is applied vertically, starting at the root of the lip and working outward to the lip border. This necessitates a high level of expertise, experience, and understanding of the underlying anatomy.

Furthermore, if you want to try out a pair of Russian lips, it is crucial to keep in mind that it is best to start with a clean slate; this means that any prior lip fillers will need to be dissolved 2 weeks ahead of time. This guarantees that the volume injected is concentrated solely in the middle of the lips. (Note: if you already have Russian lip fillers and are touching up and/or adding to them, dissolving does not apply.) (**Figs. 8–10**).

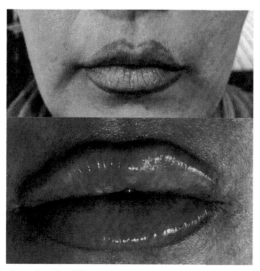

Fig. 8. Russian technique for lipofilling.

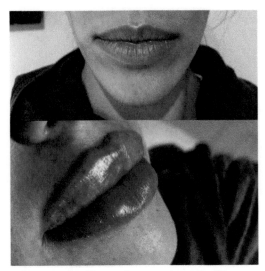

Fig. 9. Combination of Russian lip filler and conventional lip filler.

What is the difference between standard technique and Russian lip filler technique?
So, what is the difference between traditional lip filling technique and Russian lip filling technique? Standard lip fillers are typically injected horizontally into the lip, resulting in a uniform distribution of volume and fullness. To do the Russian filler procedure, however, your provider will use a smaller syringe and inject little amounts of filler vertically, concentrating on the middle of the lips. Another significant distinction is that the Russian lip filler procedure seeks to heighten the lip by focusing on the center, rather than adding overall plumpness to the lips, resulting in a heart-shaped appearance.

Additionally, due to the precision required to fill only a specific section of the lips, your Russian treatment may take longer than a conventional lip filler appointment. The surgery can take anywhere from 30 minutes to an hour, and there may be some bruising and swelling afterward, which is perfectly normal and transitory. Your supplier will be able to give you an exact schedule for how long your Russian lips will stay; but in general, they will last as long as conventional lip fillers, which is anywhere from 6 to 12 months. Accurate evaluation of the white and red rolls, Cupid's

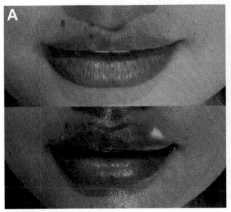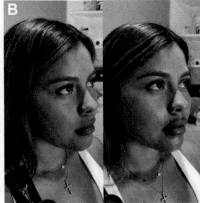

Fig. 10. (*A*) Russian lipofilling (frontal view). (*B*) Russian lipofilling (sagittal view).

bow arc, philtrum, and gingival show can help the injector determine the appropriate augmentation for each patient. In this regularly performed cosmetic surgery, tailoring therapy to lip contour, projection, and/or augmentation can produce predictable and repeatable results.

What are some side effects of Russian lips?

Although lip fillers may seem to be an easy "lunchtime treatment," it is crucial to note that they are a process with hazards. If the correct procedure is not performed correctly, major problems can arise, resulting in long-term (even permanent) damage. An increase in the number of untrained injectors offering treatments has occurred. Asymmetry, infections, and even tissue death can occur if filler is administered incorrectly. Bulging and torn lip skin, uneven and lumpy lips, and allergic responses are some of the other negative effects. Patients should also be aware that not all fillers are created equal. In truth, there are numerous distinctions across the market.

PRACTICE POINTS

HA fillers are approved by the US Food and Drug Administration for lip augmentation and/or treatment of perioral rhytides in adults 21 years and older.

Most of the complications associated with HA lip aumentation are mild and transient and can be include:

1. Injection site reaction such as pain ,erythema,and edema and vascular occlusion.
2. Combination treatment with dermal fillers and neurotoxins may demonstrate effects that last longer than either modality alone without additional adverse events.[10,14]

SUMMARY

Smile is a crucial and defining element of the face in facial proportion, and it has an enormous impact utmost the importance in the perception of feelings. Lip is perfectly perceived smile by the innovative technique will enhance the approach of the smile improvement.

CLINICS CARE POINTS

- Side effects of lip augmentation are temporary and mild, They may include: Bleeding from injection site.
- Swelling and bruising (Arnica cream or gel and ice pack are highly recommended).
- Redness and tenderness (NSAID can be prescribed to palliative the pain).
- Activation of coldsore or fever blister.
- Lip assymetry (it needs touch up after 10 days or enzyme for disolving).
- Lumps and irregularities.
- The more serious is vascular occlusion ,that needs immidiate regimen (Aspiration and microcannula blunt tip ,temporary and biodegradable product ,massage with any topical 2% nitroglycerin paste can be beneficial and stimulate quick vasodilation and should be applied each 2 hours in injection site).

AUTHORSHIP

All authors meet the International Committee of Medical Journal Editors (ICMJE) authorship criteria and are responsible for the completeness of the study. They ensure that this document is not published elsewhere in the same format in other languages, including English or electronic.

DECLARATION OF COMPETING INTEREST

We hereby declare that there are no conflicts of interest concerning this article.

CONSENT FOR PUBLICATION

All authors, give their consent for the publication of identifiable details, which can include photograph(s) and/or videos and/or case history and/or details within the text ("Material") to be published in the above Journal and Article.

REFERENCES

1. Maloney BP. Aesthetic surgery of the lip. In: Papel ID, editor. Facial plastic and reconstructive surgery. 2nd edition. New York: Thieme Medical Publishers; 2002. p. 344–52.
2. Loos BM, Maas CS. Relevant anatomy for botulinum toxin facial rejuvenation. Facial Plast Surg Clin North Am 2003;11(4):439–44.
3. Neuber F. Fat translation. Chir Kongr Verhandl Dsch Gesellch Chir 1893;20:66–8.
4. Al-Hoqail RA, Abdel Meguid EM. The lip: a histologic and analytical approach of relevance to esthetic plastic surgery. J Craniofac Surg 2009;20(3):726–32.
5. Niamtu J. Rejuvenation of the lip and perioral areas. In: Bell WH, Guerroro CA, editors. Distraction osteogenesisof the facial skeleton. Ontario (Canada): BC Decker Inc; 2007. p. 38–48.
6. Tansatit T, Apinuntrum P, Phetudom T. A typical pattern of the labial arteries with implication for lip augmentationwith injectable fillers. Aesthetic Plast Surg 2014; 38:1083–9.
7. Sadick NS, Karcher C, Palmisano L. Cosmetic dermatologyof the aging face. Clin Dermatol 2009;27(suppl):S3–12.
8. Ali MJ, Ende K, Mass CS. Perioral rejuvenation and lip augmentation. Facial Plast Surg Clin North Am 2007;15:491–500.
9. Chien AL, Qi J, Cheng N, et al. Perioral wrinkles are associated with female gender, aging, and smoking: development of a gender-specific photonumeric scale. J Am Acad Dermatol 2016;74:924–30.
10. Iblher N, Stark GB, Penna V. The aging perioral region— do we really know what is happening? J Nutr Health Aging 2012;16:581–5.
11. Segall L, Ellis DA. Therapeutic options for lip augmentation. Facial Plast Surg Clin North Am 2007;15(4):485–90.
12. Simonacci F, Bertozzi N, Grieco MP, et al. Procedure, applications, and outcomes of autologous fat grafting. Ann Med Surg (Lond) 2017;20:49–60.
13. Emsen IM. A new and different lip augmentation material containing cartilage-nous tissues harvested from rhinoplasty. J Craniofac Surg 2021;32(1):e27–8.
14. Sarnoff DS, Gotkin RH. Six steps to the "perfect" lip. J Drugs Dermatol 2012;11: 1081–8.

Lip Lift Techniques in Smile Design

Hamid Reza Fallahi, DDS, OMFS[a], Seied Omid Keyhan, DDS, OMFS[a,b],
Behnam Bohluli, DDS, OMFS[c], Behzad Cheshmi, DDS[a,*], Parastoo Jafari, DDS, MSc[d]

KEYWORDS

• Lip lift • Subnasal lip lift • Endonasal lip lift • Upper lip • Smile design

KEY POINTS

• The lips are the main aesthetic component of the facial lower third and simultaneously a substantial element for an ideally perceived smile.
• In general, the greater height of the upper vermilion has been stated to be more desirable both in male and female subjects.
• There is an experimental consensus that a greater vermilion show, short philtrum, symmetric and prominent philtral columns are aesthetically more attractive.
• Considering the condition of the anatomical structures adjacent to the lip area, such as the nasal complex, is critical in designing a treatment plan.
• Lip lift procedure can significantly affect lower nasal esthetics by decreasing the nasolabial angle and contributing to pseudo-projection of the nasal tip.

INTRODUCTION

The lips are the main aesthetic component of the facial lower third[1] and simultaneously a substantial element for an ideally perceived smile.[2] Delicate lips and well-proportioned teeth are the 2 main components of an attractive smile that are thoroughly considered in smile design.[3] One of the most accepted and common procedures that is widely used to enhance the shape and contours of the upper lip is the lip lift. Lip lift is a procedure that can effectively shorten the distance between the nasal base and the vermilion border of the upper lift through excision on the skin and the advancement of the soft tissue complex.[4] This surgical procedure has been commonly used since the 1980s for the reduction of cutaneous lip height and the establishment of a more youthful facial appearance.[5–7] The primary bullhorn lip lift was described over 4 decades ago[8] and has been consolidated as the most accepted technique. To hide the scar

Funding information: The authors received no financial support for the research, authorship, and/ or publication of this article.
[a] Maxillofacial Surgery & Implantology & Biomaterial Research Foundation, Tehran, Iran;
[b] Department of Oral & Maxillofacial Surgery, College of Medicine, Jacksonville, FL, USA; [c] Oral and Maxillofacial Surgery, University of Toronto, 124 Edward Street, Toronto, Ontario M5G 1G6, Canada; [d] Private Practice
* Corresponding author:
E-mail address: Beh.cheshomi@gmail.com

alongside the nasal base and for the removal of upper lip skin, a curvy incision is performed along the nasal sill and alar creases. The subnasal lip lift simultaneously decreases the height of the upper lip and prolabium and increases the height of the upper vermilion[9] that leads to a form that more ideally resembles the aesthetic criteria.[6] Several modifications of this procedure have been introduced.[5,10–13] Also, multiple variations have been presented to specifically address the philtrum,[11,14] lateralize subunits,[15] conceal scars,[10] or minimize excisions.[16]

DISCUSSION
Anatomy

The upper lip comprises various anatomic components. The upper lip trilaminar infrastructure has a median underlying substructural layer that is contained of the superior portion of the orbicularis oris and some bilateral contributions from the buccinators and lip elevator muscles. Multifold minor salivary glands are juxtaposed in the orbicularis oris adjacent to the mucosa. The subcutaneous fat layer underneath the skin of the upper lip contains several sweat and sebaceous glands. The upper lip exterior layer is split up into the skin and the vermilion. The red vermilion is a transitional area with a large underlying network of capillaries extended from oral mucosa toward the skin at the wet-dry line that contains an epithelium layer without glandular tissue. The philtrum is the medial portion of the upper lip that is inscribed by philtral columns bilaterally (**Fig. 1**). The cutaneous upper lip at the inferior border is confined by the vermilion; the superior border is confined by the nasal sill and alar base, and the nasolabial fold and commissures confine the lip on each lateral side. The medial aesthetic subunit of the upper lip includes the philtral grooves; additionally, each lateral aesthetic subunit comprises a philtral column and a lateral portion of lip reaching to the nasolabial folds.[17] Several anatomic criteria, including philtral distance, cupid's bow depth, and labial distance, should be measured for the procedure of lip lift preoperatively.[18]

SEX-SPECIFIC CHARACTERISTICS OF LIPS

The overall upper lip height from supramentale to stomion (23.6 vs 20.6 mm) as well as the cutaneous skin to vermilion ratio is measured to be larger in male subjects.

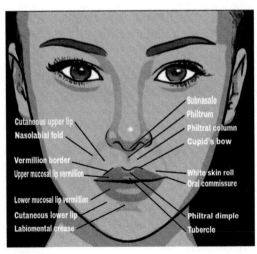

Fig. 1. Lip complex anatomy.

However, upper incisor show in female subjects is greater in comparison to male subjects (about 4 vs 2 mm, respectively).[19,20] However, some studies reported that the height of the upper vermilion is not significantly different between male and female subjects.[19,21] In general, the greater height of the upper vermilion has been stated to be more desirable in both male and female subjects.[22]

AESTHETIC IDEALS

There is an experimental consensus that a greater vermilion show, short philtrum, and symmetric and prominent philtral columns are aesthetically more attractive.[22,23] Ideally, the cutaneous skin height to upper vermilion height proportion should be less than 3.[18] Findings of studies indicated that the philtrum to upper vermilion ratio should ideally range between 2 and 2.9 and upper to lower vermilion between 0.75 and 0.8.[18,24] Consideration of these ideal ratios during the treatment planning will significantly improve lip lift outcomes.

SUBJECT'S DEMANDS
Enlargement of the Upper Lip

Findings of related studies indicate that the upper to lower lip ideal ratio is about 1.0:1.6. However, based on several factors, such as age, race, and personal preference, this ratio may slightly vary. For this reason, to achieve a more attractive appearance of the facial lower third, numerous subjects desire upper lip enlargement.

Shortness of Philtrum

A long philtrum leads to insufficient tooth show, disproportionation of facial components, and misapprehension of expressions because this situation can make subjects seem older or angrier. Ideally, the length of philtrum should range between 11 and 13 mm for female subjects and 13 and 15 mm for male subjects. However, the optimal length for philtrum must be proportionally determined in relation to other facial features of a subject.

Improvement of Teeth Show

Inadequate teeth show during smiling can occasionally cause a less passionate smile. It also makes subjects seem older than their actual age.

Cupid's Bow Contouring

A distinctly contoured cupid's bow is considered an elegant characteristic for the smile that is commonly desired by subjects. The cupid's bow can be prominently enhanced by lifting a certain portion of the lip.

Correction of Aesthetic Proportions

The facial lower third and particularly lips are not aesthetically isolated elements, instead, are an ingredient of a bigger complex that needs to be evaluated comprehensively. In other words, the outcomes of an aesthetic procedure on the lower third of the face and specifically on the lips will be pleasant and acceptable only if the modifications are planned in proportion to the other components of the face.[25]

PREOPERATIVE CONSIDERATIONS

Like any other facial aesthetic surgical procedure, proper selection of subjects and preoperative evaluation are substantial in order to achieve the best outcomes. In order to achieve the desired outcomes, various factors, such as underlying bony anatomy, cephalometric features, philtral height, vermilion height, teeth show, commissure position, fullness, and height of lower lip vermilion, and possible asymmetries should be evaluated preoperatively. Generally, because bony hard tissue has a foundational role for its overlying soft tissue, the condition of hard tissue can exacerbate or neutralize the results of procedures performed on soft tissue. The vertical maxillary excess (VME) in long face subjects and the vertical maxillary deficiency (in short face subjects) can cause excessive incisal show and shortage of incisal show, respectively. It should be noted that maxillary protrusion (SNA the angle between the sella/nasion plane and the nasion/A plane >82°) can aggravate the appearance of decreased upper lip height.

These measurements must be made individually and in proportion to each other and to other facial aesthetic components, such as the height of the facial lower third, projection of the chin, nasal tip projection, nasolabial angle, and alar base width. The bimanual traction of the upper lip tissue can be performed to estimate the approximate amount of skin to be excised and visualize the postoperative result.[10]

Considering the condition of the anatomic structures adjacent to the lip area, such as the nasal complex, is critical in designing a treatment plan. For instance, subjects with a wide alar base may require a more prominent lift in lateral segments by extending the incisions to the perialar creases, whereas subjects with a narrow alar base commonly require the lift at the central portion. For this purpose, to prevent insufficient lifting of the lateral portion, the ratio of nasal base to lip width should be reduced to 1:2.[26] Given that there is a possibility of scarring following lip lift, giving consultation to the patient in this regard and furthermore drawing the possible scarring line for the patient can prevent unexpected postoperative dissatisfaction.

A comprehensive consultation regarding procedural details, recovery stages, potential complications, and most importantly, shared decision making pertinent to the patient's desires is among the major points in the preoperative phase.

GENERAL PROCEDURAL APPROACH
Measuring

The most critical index that must be carefully measured is the amount of skin that must be excised in each area of the cutaneous lip. After cleaning the surgical field with a chlorhexidine wipe, the patient is moved to the supine position. Important points, such as the base and center of the columella, are marked using a fine marker. At this point, the distance from the columellar base to the cupid's bow base is measured using a caliper to determine the current length of the philtrum. The measurements should be taken on the skin in a resting condition, and the skin of the area should not be in a stretched form. Then, by returning the patient to a sitting position, various indicators, such as upper to lower red lip proportion, the amount of the teeth show, the philtrum length, and the possible asymmetries, are evaluated so that appropriate marking can be made based on these criteria.

Marking

The points spotted in the measurement step should be connected using a marker. Marking in the supine position begins by outlining of the nasal base. Vertical lines at the philtral columns and alar bases can be drawn as guidelines to avoid asymmetric marking and incisions. The incisions should be extended laterally to the points where the outer alar contours transition from curved to vertical. Also, the incisions will be continued medially following the alar bending, along the sill base, and in the direction of the base of the columella. The nasal sill should not be overstepped. If asymmetry is observed, the markings should be done asymmetrically to the same extent so that at the time of excisions, the appropriate amount of tissue is removed from each side and the asymmetries are eliminated. Finally, the markings that correspond to the authors' treatment plan and set up of the outcomes are shown to the patient to examine her/his judgment.

SURGICAL TECHNIQUE

Anesthetic solution (Lidocaine HCl 2% and Epinephrine 1:100,000) is injected into the gingivolabial sulcus bilaterally. Following needle renewal, the anesthetic solution should also be injected into the nasal base, alar corners, nasal sill, and the lower aspects of the cutaneous lip. The skin adjacent to the surgical site should be prepared with povidone-iodine. Skin incisions are made using a no. 15c blade beginning from the nasal base. After making the upper incision from one side to the other, the lower

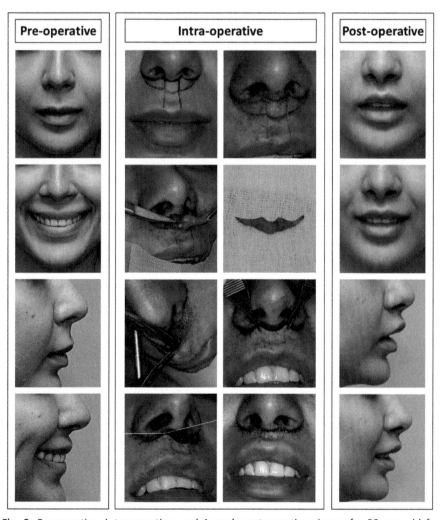

Fig. 2. Preoperative, intraoperative, and 1-week postoperative views of a 28-year-old female patient who underwent lip lift using conventional technique.

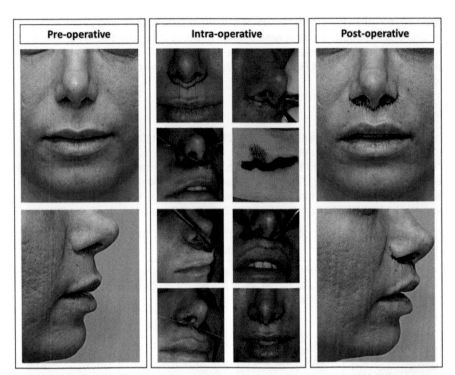

Fig. 3. Preoperative, intraoperative, and immediate postoperative views of a 34-year-old female patient who underwent lip lift using conventional technique.

incision is completed accordingly. The excision's depth should be within the subcutaneous tissues so that the vessels are detected. Invasion of deeper tissues may cause damage to the vessels, which can result in exacerbation of edema postoperatively. In order to minimize any functional consequences, impinging of the muscles should be avoided as much as possible. Hemostasis in the surgical site can be established using bipolar cautery and oxymetazoline-soaked gauzes. To minimize tension along the wound margins, the flap should be detached and lifted as far as possible from the underlying muscles. A delicate skin hook can be used to minimize tissue damage. A no. 15c blade should be used mediolaterally 1 to 2 cm inferior to the lower margin of incision to prepare a uniform thickness flap. Suturing should begin from the medial portion using a 5-0 Monocryl thread and a tapered needle to obtain a properly deep fixation. Attention must be taken to avoid shortening of the nasal sill height. Subsequently, a 6-0 Prolene suture with a tapered needle should be used in a simple interrupted fashion on the skin, and furthermore, to augment lip eversion, a vertical mattress can be used at the sill area, or just lateral to it (**Figs. 2–4**).

Postoperative Care

Patients should apply antibiotic ointment to the excision area for 1 week postoperatively. Showering should be postponed for at least 2 days after surgery. Because swelling is one of the most common short-term complications after surgery, informing patients about it can reduce their anxiety. Avoiding intense activities in addition to keeping the head elevated and applying cool compresses can significantly help minimize edema postoperatively. The use of thin tape strips after the removal of the

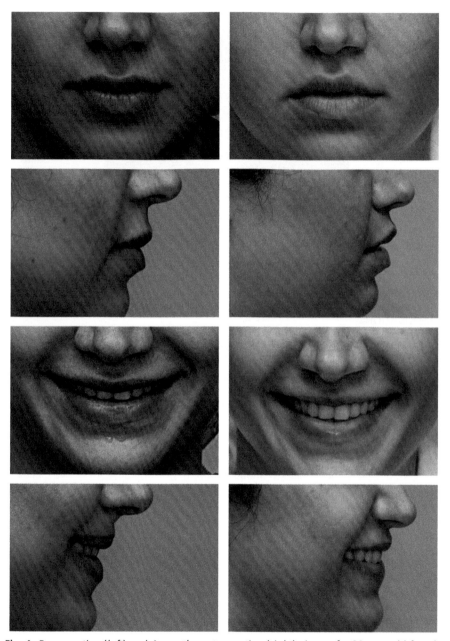

Fig. 4. Preoperative (*left*) and 4-month postoperative (*right*) views of a 39-year-old female patient who underwent lip lift using conventional technique.

sutures can help support the soft tissue of the incision area. Avoiding direct exposure to sunlight by applying sunscreen for at least a year can help speed up the healing process of incision lines. In case the process of scar healing in the area is prolonged, adjuvant methods, such as dermabrasion and laser therapy, can also be used (**Fig. 5**).

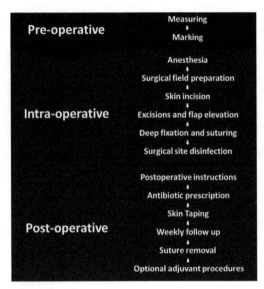

Fig. 5. General procedural flowchart.

COMPLICATIONS

Scarring is generally the patient's main concern and has been reported in 1% to 5% of cases.[10,11] A precise surgical technique, delicate handling of tissues, and precise apposition of the flap can be helpful in minimizing scarring. Wound breakdown is the second most common complication associated with the dehiscence of the skin in the area, which can be managed using common scar revision techniques. Asymmetry, overcorrection, and undercorrection are among the other most common potential complications of lip lift. Obviously, the management of undercorrection is simpler and more feasible than overcorrection adjustment. Thus, it is necessary to observe maximum delicacy and accuracy in designing the treatment plan and surgical process, especially in subjects with VME or significant teeth show. Intraoperative or postoperative excessive bleeding owing to preexisting blood disorders, hematoma, infections, which can be commonly prevented via antibiotics prescription, and ecchymosis or bruising are also among the potential complications of this procedure. The risk of distortions in the alar base area is higher with the endonasal technique[10]; however, it can also occur in cases of large lifting and intense tension across the margins of incisions. The subnasal lip lift method mainly addresses the central portion of the upper lip and provides lower levels of effectiveness in lateral parts. This deficiency is more notable in cases with a narrower width of alar base. The shape and form of the philtrum can significantly impact the procedure's outcome. Central insertion of philtral columns in a nonparallel manner can be used to lateralize the insertion of columns and reduce the upper lip height.[27] Postoperative hypoesthesia and paresthesia are rare. However, they can occur following profound dissections close to the muscle. Eversion of the upper lip is one of the natural consequences of a lip lift, which causes a portion of the inner wet red lip to be exposed to air now more than before. Adapting to this new condition may take some time for patients.

LITERATURE REVIEW

Because of the variety of deficiencies and differences in patients' desires, various lip lift techniques with diverse applications have been introduced so far. Each of these

Table 1
Lip lift techniques[7]

	Author(s), Ref., Year	Method/Title	Schematic View
Direct lip lift	Meyer & Kesselring,[28] 1976	Upper and lower lip	
Indirect lip lift	Cardoso & Sperli,[29] 1971	Bullhorn subnasal lip lift	
	Austin,[11] 1986	Philtrum stretching subtype I	
	Austin,[11] 1986	Philtrum stretching subtype II	
	González-Ulloa,[14] 1979	L-shaped philtrum lift	
	Brenda,[15] 1994	Extended incision	
	Greenwald,[30] 1985	Greenwald incision	
	Cardim et al,[31] 2011	Double duck suspension	
	Santanchè & Bonarrigo,[32] 2004	Italian technique	

(continued on next page)

Table 1
(continued)

	Author(s), Ref., Year	Method/Title	Schematic View
Corner of the mouth lift	Greenwald,[30] 1985	Lentoid incision	
	Austin & Weston,[33] 1994	Triangular incision	
	Perkins,[34] 2007	Rhomboidal incision	
	Ching & Flowers,[35] 2005	Valentine anguloplasty	
	Parsa et al,[36] 2010	Extended incision	
	Borges,[37] 1989	Lentoid excision for correction of "sad pleats"	
Nonscar lip lift	Echo et al,[16] 2011	Nonscar suspension technique	

techniques has its own strengths, weaknesses, and limitations. Moragas and colleagues[7] in a systematic review study comprehensively evaluated the lip lift techniques (**Table 1**).

A lip lift procedure can significantly affect lower nasal esthetics by decreasing the nasolabial angle and contributing to pseudoprojection of the nasal tip.[38] Incision designs in some surgical techniques, such as endonasal lip lifts,[10] have involved nasal caudal structures. The most serious disadvantage of this technique is nasal sill disruption, which can be minimized by using high accuracy during surgery (**Fig. 6**).

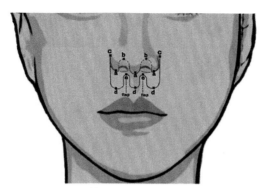

Fig. 6. Endonasal lip lift technique.[10] A: Alar/columellar base, B: key suture location, C: superolateral tip of resection, D: flap base, E: flap apex.

Moreover, concomitant open rhinoplasty and upper lip lift have recently been introduced by Bessler.[39] The upper lip length can have a significant influence on the aesthetic proportions of nasal appearance, particularly, on the projection of the nasal tip. Therefore, this combination is indicated in cases that the length of the upper lip may exceed the planned degree of nasal tip projection (**Fig. 7**).

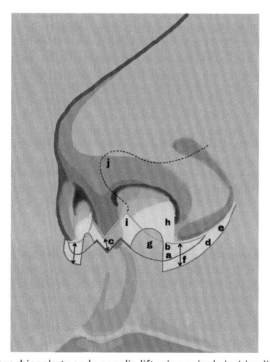

Fig. 7. Simultaneous rhinoplasty and upper lip lift using a single incision line. (a) The caudal IL of SLL (*dark blue*); (b) cranial IL of SLL (*light blue*); (c) the craniocaudal dimension of medial skin resection; (d) the caudal IL of ELL (*dark green*); (e) the cranial IL of ELL (*lime green*); (f) the craniocaudal dimension of lateral skin resection; (g) the endonasal skin flap; (h) the recipient site for endonasal skin flap; (i) the medial crus posterior portion (*dotted line*); (j) the marginal incision for the open rhinoplasty.[39] IL, incision line ELL, endonasal lip lift; SLL, subnasal lip lift.

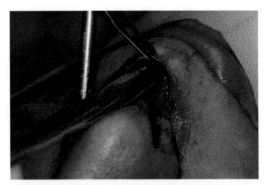

Fig. 8. Elevation of deep-plane sub-SMAS over the muscle layer.

Talei[40] has developed a modified lip lift technique that focuses on releasing the superficial musculoaponeurotic system (SMAS) in the patient's lip area. This technique can mainly be applied in combination with a facelift procedure. Deep releasing of the SMAS in the upper lip area can provide a tension-free suspension to the nasal base ligaments. In addition, deep suspension suturing of the tissue results in convenient healing in this high-risk dynamic area (**Fig. 8**).

Female and male subjects have usually diverse facial characteristics that result in feminine and masculine appearance, respectively. The lips, as well, are the main aesthetic component of the facial lower third that strongly imply gender-specific features. The procedure of lip lift reduces the nasal base to the vermilion border distance via cutaneous excisions and advancement of tissues. Although lip lift frequently causes subtle change, these adjustments can intentionally feminize the facial appearance.[4]

Drooping of the lip corners in the perioral region can create a "sad mouth" appearance in patients. This condition often needs to be addressed directly owing to the fact that the use of more general techniques, such as facelift, is not able to properly eliminate this problem.[41] Corner of lip lift is the surgical technique introduced to refine this miss-expression, establishing a cheerful appearance. This procedure is rarely used independently but is often used in combination with the conventional subnasal lip lift technique especially in cases with elongated cutaneous upper lip and limited dental show.[13]

SUMMARY

The lips are the main aesthetic component of the facial lower third and simultaneously a substantial element for an ideally perceived smile. One of the most accepted and common procedures that is widely used to enhance the shape and contours of the upper lip is the lip lift. Patients desire a conservative, permanent, and effective solution for the enhancement of their lips, and lip lift has been shown to be able to meet these demands. With a careful treatment plan and professional surgery, a lip lift can reliably be used for the reduction of the philtrum height, enlargement of the upper vermilion, improvement of the dental show, restoration of facial aesthetic proportions, and creation of an enchanting smile.

CLINICS CARE POINTS

- The lips are the main aesthetic component of the facial lower third and simultaneously a substantial element for an ideally perceived smile.

- The lips, as well, are the main aesthetic component of the facial lower third that strongly implies gender-specific features. Upper incisor show in female subjects is greater in comparison to male subjects.
- A greater vermilion show, short philtrum, and symmetric and prominent philtral columns are aesthetically more attractive.
- In order to achieve the desired outcomes, various factors, such as underlying bony anatomy, cephalometric features, philtral height, vermilion height, teeth show, commissure position, fullness, and height of lower lip vermilion, and possible asymmetries should be evaluated preoperatively.
- The most critical index that must be carefully measured is the amount of skin that must be excised in each area of the cutaneous lip.
- The excision's depth should be within the subcutaneous tissues so that the vessels are detected. Invasion of deeper tissues may cause damage to the vessels, which can result in exacerbation of edema postoperatively. In order to minimize any functional consequences, impinging of the muscles should be avoided as much as possible.
- In case the process of scar healing in the area is prolonged, adjuvant methods, such as dermabrasion and laser therapy, can also be used.
- A precise surgical technique, delicate handling of tissues, and precise apposition of the flap can be helpful in minimizing scarring.
- Lip lift procedure can significantly affect lower nasal esthetics by decreasing the nasolabial angle and contributing to pseudo-projection of the nasal tip.
- Concomitant open rhinoplasty and upper lip lift have recently been introduced by Bessler.[39]
- The modified lip lift technique that focuses on releasing the superficial musculoaponeurotic system can mainly be applied in combination with a facelift procedure.
- Corner of lip lift is the surgical technique introduced to refine "sad mouth" appearance, establishing a cheerful appearance.

SUMMARY

Patients desire a conservative, permanent, and effective solution for the enhancement of their lips, and lip lift has been shown to be able to meet these demands. With a careful treatment plan and professional surgery, a lip lift can reliably be used for the reduction of the philtrum height, enlargement of the upper vermilion, improvement of the dental show, restoration of facial aesthetic proportions, and creation of an enchanting smile.

COMPETING INTERESTS

The authors declare that they have no competing interests.

REFERENCES

1. Fallahi HR, Zandian D, Cheshmi B, et al. Facial analysis and clinical evaluation charts. integrated procedures in facial cosmetic surgery. Springer; 2021. p. 35–58.
2. Thomas M, D'Silva J, Kohli S, et al. Lip designing: the need for a beautiful smile: an Indian perspective. Indian J Dental Res 2014;25(4):449.
3. Coachman C, Calamita MA, Sesma N. Dynamic documentation of the smile and the 2D/3D digital smile design process. Int J Periodontics Restorative Dent 2017; 37(2):183–93.

4. Salibian AA, Bluebond-Langner R. Lip lift. Facial Plast Surg Clin 2019;27(2): 261–6.

5. Mommaerts MY, Blythe JN. Rejuvenation of the ageing upper lip and nose with suspension lifting. J Cranio-Maxillofacial Surg 2016;44(9):1123–5.

6. Lee DE, Hur SW, Lee JH, et al. Central lip lift as aesthetic and physiognomic plastic surgery: the effect on lower facial profile. Aesthet Surg J 2015;35(6):698–707.

7. Moragas JSM, Vercruysse HJ, Mommaerts MY. Non-filling" procedures for lip augmentation: a systematic review of contemporary techniques and their outcomes. J Cranio-Maxillofacial Surg 2014;42(6):943–52.

8. Stack G. Transactions of the fifth international congress of plastic and reconstructive surgery. Thousand Oaks, CA: SAGE Publications Sage CA; 1972.

9. Penna V, Iblher N, Bannasch H, et al. Proving the effectiveness of the lip lift for treatment of the aging lip: a morphometric evaluation. Plast Reconstr Surg 2010;126(2):83e-4e.

10. Raphael P, Harris R, Harris SW. The endonasal lip lift: personal technique. Aesthet Surg J 2014;34(3):457–68.

11. Austin HW. The lip lift. Plast Reconstr Surg 1986;77(6):990–4.

12. Li YK, Ritz M. The modified bull's horn upper lip lift. J Plast Reconstr Aesthet Surg 2018;71(8):1216–30.

13. Weston GW, Poindexter BD, Sigal RK, et al. Lifting lips: 28 years of experience using the direct excision approach to rejuvenating the aging mouth. Aesthet Surg J 2009;29(2):83–6.

14. González-Ulloa M. The aging upper lip. Ann Plast Surg 1979;2(4):299–303.

15. Brenda E. Lifting of the upper lip using a single extensive incision. Br J Plast Surg 1994;47(1):50–3.

16. Echo A, Momoh AO, Yuksel E. The no-scar lip-lift: upper lip suspension technique. Aesthetic Plast Surg 2011;35(4):617–23.

17. Lewin JM, Carucci JA. Staged flaps. Reconstructive Dermatologic Surgery; 2018. p. 119.

18. Raphael P, Harris R, Harris SW. Analysis and classification of the upper lip aesthetic unit. Plast Reconstr Surg 2013;132(3):543–51.

19. Anic-Milosevic S, Mestrovic S, Prlić A, et al. Proportions in the upper lip–lower lip–chin area of the lower face as determined by photogrammetric method. J Cranio-Maxillofacial Surg 2010;38(2):90–5.

20. Farkas LG, Katic M, Hreczko TA, et al. Anthropometric proportions in the upper lip-lower lip-chin area of the lower face in young white adults. Am J Orthod 1984;86(1):52–60.

21. Fernández-Riveiro P, Suárez-Quintanilla D, Smyth-Chamosa E, et al. Linear photogrammetric analysis of the soft tissue facial profile. Am J Orthod Dentofacial Orthop 2002;122(1):59–66.

22. Penna V, Fricke A, Iblher N, et al. The attractive lip: a photomorphometric analysis. J Plast Reconstr Aesthet Surg 2015;68(7):920–9.

23. Suryadevara AC. Update on perioral cosmetic enhancement. Curr Opin Otolaryngol Head Neck Surg 2008;16(4):347–51.

24. Perkins SW, Sandel IVHD. Anatomic considerations, analysis, and the aging process of the perioral region. Facial Plast Surg Clin North America 2007;15(4): 403–7.

25. Linkov G. Update on upper lip lift. Adv Cosmet Surg, E-Book 2021;2021:207.

26. Waldman SR. The subnasal lift. Facial Plast Surg Clin North America 2007;15(4): 513–6.

27. Georgiou CA, Benatar M, Bardot J, et al. Morphologic variations of the philtrum and their effect in the upper lip lift. Plast Reconstr Surg 2014;134(6):996e-7e.

28. Meyer R, Kesselring UK. Aesthetic surgery in the perioral region. Aesthet Plast Surg 1976;1(1):61–9.

29. Rhytidoplasty of the upper lip. In: Cardoso A, Sperli A, editors. Transactions of the fifth international congress of plastic and reconstructive surgery. Butterworth and Co Melbourne; 1971.

30. Greenwald AE. The lip lift cheilopexy for cheiloptosis. Am J Cosmet Surg 1985; 2(1):16–23.

31. Cardim VLN, Silva AdS, Salomons RL, et al. Double duck" nasolabial lifting. Revista Brasileira de Cirurgia Plástica 2011;26:466–71.

32. Santanchè P, Bonarrigo C. Lifting of the upper lip: personal technique. Plast Reconstr Surg 2004;113(6):1828–35.

33. Austin HW, Weston GW. Rejuvenating the aging mouth. Perspect Plast Surg 1994;8(01):27–56.

34. Perkins SW. The corner of the mouth lift and management of the oral commissure grooves. Facial Plast Surg Clin North America 2007;15(4):471–6.

35. Ching S, Flowers R, editors. Perioral rejuvenation using the valentine anguloplasty. American Society for Aesthetic Plastic Surgery Annual Meeting; 2005.

36. Parsa FD, Parsa NN, Murariu D. Surgical correction of the frowning mouth. Plast Reconstr Surg 2010;125(2):667–76.

37. Borges AF. Sad pleats. Ann Plast Surg 1989;22(1):74–5.

38. Marechek A, Perenack J, Christensen BJ. Subnasal lip lift and its effect on nasal esthetics. J Oral Maxillofac Surg 2021;79(4):895–901.

39. Bessler S. Combining rhinoplasty with upper lip–lift using a single incision line. JAMA Facial Plast Surg 2018;20(2):166–7.

40. Talei B. The modified upper lip lift: advanced approach with deep-plane release and secure suspension: 823-patient series. Facial Plast Surg Clin 2019;27(3): 385–98.

41. Clevens RA, Khelemsky R, Sayal NR. The corner of lip lift technique. Facial Plast Surg Aesthet Med 2020;22(5):389–90.

Contemporary Smile Design: An Orthodontic Perspective

Chung How Kau, BDS, MScD, MBA, PhD, MOrth, FDSGlas, FDSEdin, FFDIre, FICD, ABO*,
Terpsithea Christou, DDS, MS, ABO, Shubam Sharma, BDS, MPH

KEYWORDS

- Smile esthetics • Smile design • Orthodontic appliances • 3D imaging
- Orthodontic aligners and customized 3D appliances for orthodontics

KEY POINTS

- The use of 3D technology for records and diagnostic planning.
- Bracket placement for optimum smile design.
- Aligner treatment during orthodontic treatment.
- Surgical interventions for orthodontic smile design.
- TADs for orthodontic tooth movement and tooth control.

INTRODUCTION

Orthodontists make a huge impact on the lives of people seeking better smiles. Although there are various reasons why people seek orthodontic care, one of the reasons is the ability of orthodontists to convert a malocclusion into well-balanced, pleasing, and artistic appearance of teeth within the smile framework. With this end point in mind, the goal of the orthodontist is to evaluate how a smile will fit into the facial morphology of any given individual.

In this new age of selfies and social media boom, laypeople have started noticing even the slightest asymmetries noticeable in the past only to clinicians. How a smile can be crafted into an individual's face with harmony and balance is truly important. Unconsciously, smiling is the most important nonverbal way of communication and perception. It is by far the most effective way to express emotions and create connections.[1,2] Every individual carries a unique smile to their face, and there is no perfect recipe for a smile. However, over the years, many studies have been published discussing the parameters involved in creating a perfect smile.[3,4] The goal of orthodontic treatment should be to achieve a smile that is in harmony with the face.[5]

Department of Orthodontics, School of Dentistry, University of Alabama Birmingham, Suite 305, 1919 7th Avenue South, Birmingham AL 35294, USA
* Corresponding author.
E-mail address: ckau@uab.edu

Dent Clin N Am 66 (2022) 459–475
https://doi.org/10.1016/j.cden.2022.02.007
0011-8532/22/© 2022 Elsevier Inc. All rights reserved.

dental.theclinics.com

Esthetics of a Smile

In the past, many orthodontists focused on the function and ideal rehabilitation of the dental malocclusion. In recent times, it has been found that despite attempts to finish to an ideal dental occlusion, the perception of the smile was found to be less than perfect. In fact, a recent study found that of the 68 occlusal finishes for the American Board of Orthodontics examination, only 2 of the finished results were deemed to have a perfect smile by a panel of judges.[6] This same sample was further validated by a panel of judges of different ethnic background, and similar results were achieved.[7] These finding reexamined the occlusal goals of treatment and highlighted the perceptive effect that needs to be brought about during treatment.

Although many analyses and many studies have discussed the variables that define a good smile, it is universally accepted that the following components are important: (1) smile arc projection,[8] buccal corridor display,[9] and amount of gingival exposure at smiling[10]; (2) presence of gingival and incisal asymmetry[1]; (3) presence of midline shift and changes in axial proclination[11]; and (4) maxillary incisors ratio, size, and symmetry.[12]

Vertical positioning of the upper incisors helps in achieving a younger and dynamic smile. The incisal edge of maxillary central incisors must be below the cuspid tip of canines, ensuring dominance of the central incisors.[13] The step between central and lateral incisors should range from 1.0 to 1.5 mm for women and from 0.5 to 1.0 mm for men.[13]

How a smile is viewed is also important. For example, when viewing from frontal photographs, the downward positioning of maxillary plane and head inclination can lead to greater exposure of the incisors. On the other hand, upward positioning of the maxillary plane and head inclination can lead to less exposure of the upper incisors thereby hindering the original smile.[14] On smiling, the width and height ratios for the maxillary central incisors should be 75% to 85%.[15] Symmetric incisal edges are also very important in keeping good esthetics. If the lateral incisors are too narrow or thin, interdisciplinary treatment options should be considered. Slightest gaps in the frontal esthetic zone can be unpleasing to look at, and all dental spacing should be closed. Any deviation of the midline equivalent to 2 mm or greater should be addressed clinically. One great way to avoid or eliminate black areas is maintaining tight contacts, modifying contact areas, and increasing the surface areas of the connectors.[11]

Many orthodontists attempt to categorize the smile into components that can be addressed. In general, the smile is made up of 3 components.

Gingival component

This component consists of 4 elements: the texture, the color, the shape, and the amount that shows on smiling. A healthy gingiva is stippled and firm, normally coral pink, but the color depends on the amount of pigmentations and the race of the subject. The ideal location of the gingiva is 3 mm above the alveolar bone crest (facially) assuring the gingival margin of the central incisor is on the same level as the canine's margin, and slightly higher than the one of the lateral incisors, with the zenith slightly to the distal of the crown's long axis of the central incisior and canine and on the long axis of the lateral incisor.[13] Also, the dental papilla normally should fill the interdental space showing no "black triangles"; furthermore, according to Kokich and colleagues[16] up to 3 mm of gingival height that shows on smile is considered acceptable.

Dental component

This component consists of 5 elements: the color, the shape, the size, the position, and the alignment.

Any decalcification, interior or exterior staining, can affect the teeth color and ultimately affect the smile esthetic because, from the patient perspective, the teeth color is one of the most important factors in smile attractiveness.[17,18] According to Heravi and colleagues,[19] the teeth shape is an essential element in creating a charming smile; people prefer the round shape compared with the triangular and square incisors. In addition, the size of the teeth was proved to be important[20]: lateral incisor size, width to height ratio, and the crown size proportion of the anterior teeth.[21,22] Furthermore, the position of the anterior teeth in the 3D space is fundamental in designing a charming smile; vertically, the upper anterior teeth incisal edges are supposed to be in harmony with the curvature of the lower lip with ideally full exposure upon smiling.[2,4,23] However, transversely, perfect alignment with no rotations, no spacing, and with the upper dental midline coinciding with the midsagittal plane represents the optimal situation. Nonetheless, Bhuvaneswaran[24] mentions that a discrepancy up to 2 mm was unnoticeable from laypeople as long as the contact line between the upper central incisors is parallel to the facial midline. Last, the sagittal position and inclination of the upper front teeth is a major component in providing an adequate anterior guidance, providing anterior teeth exposure, and ensuring good lip support that is essential for smile esthetic.

Soft tissue component
The lips are the frame of the smile: their position, the curvature, and their thickness are vital elements for a pleasant smile. The upper lip position can be optimal showing the full crown length of upper teeth; high, revealing more than 2 mm of gingival display; or low, exposing less than 70% of the upper central incisors. Also, the curvature and the symmetry of the upper lip were found to be important parts of the smile[25]; they depend primarily on neuromuscular factors. Last, the thickness of the upper lip seems to have significant influence on the overall smile attractiveness.[26]

In summary, smile design must encompass not only straight teeth but also other factors that include size, color, gingival display, and smile drape.[6,7]

Clinical Care Points: Role of the Orthodontist

The orthodontist's role in smile design takes several forms. The following key points are important for the orthodontist to pay attention to.

Using technology to capture diagnostic records of the patient
Many tools are available for orthodontists to capture the smile. Static 2D records consisting of pictures, study models, and radiographs are the mainstay of the initial record.[27] These records should be collated into a standard composite layout for easy evaluation and treatment planning. Once these pictures are captured, a goal-oriented method can carefully map out to complete the end goal of the treatment plan (**Fig. 1**). In recent years, 3D technology has helped to create spatial awareness of the skeletal structures and relationship of teeth.[28] These technologies create true visualization of the limits of tooth movement with the frame of the jaws.[29] Newer and exciting innovations archive the 3D virtual patient effectively[30,31] and simulate smile and lip movements of the soft tissue (**Fig. 2**). Surgical interventions and surgical simulation create predictable and enhanced communications between surgeons and orthodontists.[32–35] Even more advanced technologies have also incorporated the movement of the jaws in real time hence redefining dynamic positioning of the condyle and centric relation.[36,37] Finally, 3D customized appliances are now readily available to deliver the ideal treatment plan and position the teeth accurately in the smile framework (**Fig. 3**).

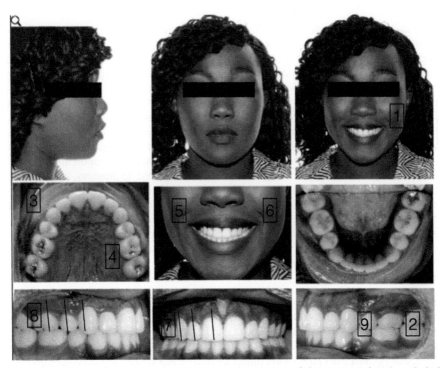

Fig. 1. Nine Composite pictures depicting the 2 dimensions of the patient's facial, smile balance, and teeth. The goals of treatment are (1) smile design within the face, (2) molar relationship, (3) alignment and (4) rotational control of teeth, (5) overbite, (6) overjet, (7) inclination, and (8) angulation of teeth and cusp to fossa interdigitation.

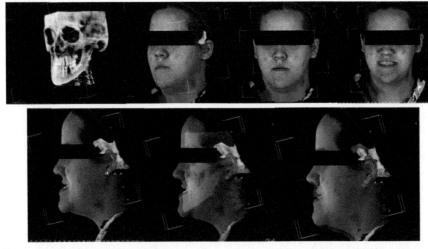

Fig. 2. 3D Imaging: A combination of surface scanning of the photographic face (in static and on smiling) and the traditional cone beam imaging technology. The 3D pictures were captured by a 3dMD Camera (3dMD LLC, Atlanta, Georgia, USA), and the Cone Beam Computed tomographies (CBCTs) are from the Carestream 9500 (Carestream, Atlanta, GA, USA) machine. These 2 types of imaging technologies are carefully combined using the 3D Vultus software (3dMD LLC, Atlanta, GA, USA). The images show that the soft tissue significantly masks the underlying skeletal structures and also depict the dynamic impact of the musculature of the smile.

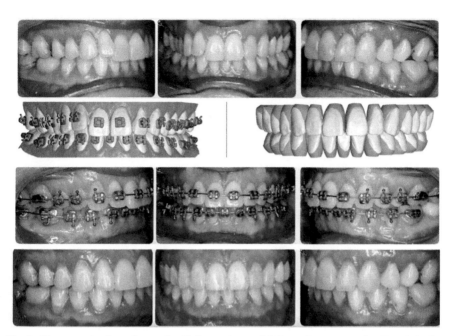

Fig. 3. 3D customized appliances by KL Owen Braces (KLOwen Braces, Austin, TX, USA). The exact position of the brackets is prescribed onto the 3D rendering to produce the desired alignment and esthetic results. Once the brackets have been set 3 dimensionally, a rubber-based transfer jig is used to indirectly bond the brackets onto the teeth. This case shows a Class IID2 malocclusion with one lower incisor missing. The treatment using customized braces took only 4 visits to complete.

Managing the gummy smile on patient with excessive gingival display

The amount of gingival display affects the perception of a smile.[6,7] There are several reasons for excessive gingival display or gummy smile. These reasons include the overgrowth of gingiva, supraeruption of upper incisors, and vertical maxillary excess. The orthodontists with the help of other dental specialties can significantly improve the gummy smile of an individual. A variety of procedures can be performed orthodontically and surgically. Gummy displays may be managed in the following 3 ways:

1. Displays within 2 to 4 mm may be managed by intruding the teeth orthodontically, crown lengthening, or Botox.
2. Displays of 4 to 8 mm may be treated by lip stabilization, or surgery can be considered.
3. Displays of more than 8 mm need to be managed with surgery alone.

Surgical management. Broadly speaking, highly distinguished or excessive gummy smiles are the result of vertical maxillary excess.[38,39] The cause of the gummy smile should first be identified as skeletal, dentoalveolar, or musculature. If a skeletal disproportion exists, the Le Fort 1 osteotomy can help reduce the maxillary excess (**Fig. 4**); it decreases the vertical skeletal length of the maxilla thereby decreasing the amount of gingiva show. These surgeries are performed under general anesthesia, and the cuts are done inside the mouth. A wedge of bone that coincides with the vertical excess is removed. These procedures must be carefully planned and facial balanced achieved

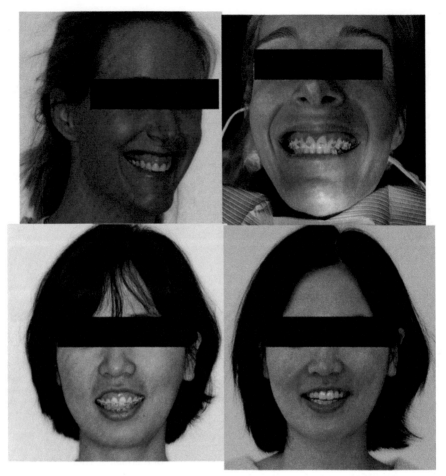

Fig. 4. Gummy smiles with more than 8 mm gingival excess for both sets of patients. Each patient received surgical vertical impactions of the maxilla up to 6 to 8 mm. The resultant smile within the smile framework was greatly improved.

to reduce unwanted facial results.[40] There is often a limit to the amount of bone that can be removed.

Botulinum type A toxin (Botox). Botulinum type A toxin (Botox) has been used in reducing the hypermobility of muscles and soft tissues associated with smiles having excessive gingival display.[41] This procedure is carried out when the muscles of the smile are overretracted. The goal of this treatment is to reduce the hyperactivity of the muscles thereby reducing the extent of the smile drape and also the gingival display. Some investigators describe measuring the length between the lower margin of upper lip and the gingival margin of upper central incisor and have seen noticeable change after using Botox. This simple procedure can be done by an orthodontist, and normally 2.5 U per 0.1 mL is injected in 2 sites on each side of the face. These points coincide anatomically with the levator labii superioris alaeque nasi, levator labii superioris (LLS), and the LLS and zygomaticus minor muscle meeting on right and left sides of the face. The Botox injection weakens the ability of the muscles to contract thus reducing the hypercontraction, which leads to lesser pull of the lip while smiling. If Botox is considered to treat the excessive gingival display due to the contraction of muscles, there should be a minimum 5 mm of gingival display to achieve pleasing results. The effects may not be long lasting, and the procedure is repeated throughout life.

Gingivectomy or apical reposition flaps. When gingival tissues are overgrown, hyperplastic, or inflamed, it creates an unesthetic appearance of the gingiva; it may also affect the ability of the patient to keep good oral hygiene. Overgrowth of gingiva in such cases can lead to a gummy smile, which if not treated in conjunction with orthodontics, can lead to poor esthetics results. Many orthodontists prefer to perform gingivectomies themselves because it saves chair time and saves on costs for the patient. The main aim is to remove excess gingival tissue, expose the underlying tooth, and create proper gingival contours. One should always be careful not to invade the natural biological width while carrying out these procedures. Gingivectomies are always preferred when there is excess amount of keratinized tissue, and the bone levels are within normal limits (**Fig. 5**). Care should be taken while taking out extra tissue only to achieve good esthetic results.[42] Apically positioned flap surgeries are performed when the gingivectomies do not suffice and are carried out in 2 scenarios: first, when the distance between CEJ and alveolar crest is normal and there is normal amount of keratinized tissue, and second, when the bone and CEJ are at same level and the keratinized tissue is within normal limits, in which case apical position flap with osseous reduction is preferred.[43] These procedures are often done by the periodontists or oral surgeons.

Orthodontic Strategies for Fixed Appliances

The mainstay in orthodontic treatment is the orthodontic bracket and wire. Each set of brackets is made up of a preadjusted system that has prescribed, or custom, 3D

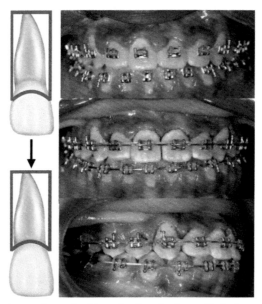

Fig. 5. Gingivectomies performed with a simple soft tissue diode laser. The goal is not to invade the biological width but at the same time exposing as much of the clinical crown as possible.

values embedded within each bracket. An orthodontic wire is placed onto the bracket slot, and the 3D angles are expressed when the bracket slot is fully expressed thereby resulting in a pleasing result for both the occlusion and smile. Traditionally, the basic goal for the placement of the brackets is the center of the clinical crown and along the long axis of the tooth. However, careful manipulation during bracket placement on the tooth can alter the tooth position and enhance the smile.

Deliberate apical positioning of the anterior orthodontic brackets

Placing brackets gingivally has been advocated by the authors and others. This simple but deliberate placement of the bracket can help to develop the smile arc that maximizes the smile within the face[1,3] (**Fig. 6**). Often, during the planning stage, the maxillary arch wire plane is planned to be parallel to the upper lip, whereas the lower lip defines the incisal edges of the upper incisors. The difference in bracket placement heights in anterior and posteriors enables the maxillary cant to increase with respect to the true smiling plane. The gingival position of the brackets produces a clockwise rotation of the anterior segment via extrusion of the upper anterior when compared with the upper premolars.[44] Bite turbos and very light elastics can help in uprighting the teeth in the initial phase on light wires.[45]

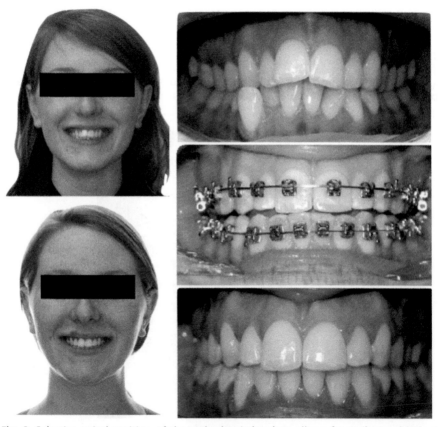

Fig. 6. Selective apical position of the orthodontic brackets allows for smile arc development. A patient who initially presented with a reverse smile arch and proclined teeth developed a final result in which a consonant smile and upright teeth are achieved.

Torque control (low torque)

A recent study has shown that the maxillary incisor can change significantly in nonextraction class I, II, and III dental malocclusions. The findings showed that in class I and III malocclusions, the incisors are proclined or tipped forward, and in class II malocclusions the teeth are more upright at the end of treatment.[46] At present, nonextraction treatment is a popular choice among patients. However, in most of these cases, the maxillary incisors are proclined and crowding is present. To counteract the unwanted flaring of the teeth, which flattens the smile, placing the brackets more gingivally on the tooth surface helps in reducing the torque that is built in the bracket. The flaring of upper incisors can also be prevented by flipping the brackets 180° on the intended tooth surface.

Interproximal reduction or addition of tooth structure

Interproximal reduction (IPR) involves deliberate removal of enamel from the contact areas of adjacent teeth. This technique creates space to allow teeth movement and allow patients to avoid extractions. IPR is done by using diamond disks, metal strips, or burs. IPR leads to changes in the size of teeth and sometimes increases tooth stability after completion of treatment. IPR can also eliminate black triangles that sometimes form due to horizontal bone loss or narrow contact areas. In other instances, where teeth are too small, careful addition of tooth-colored composites can also guide the clinician through the process of smile design. A combination of either one or both is required to produce a pleasing smile (**Fig. 7**).

Smile Design with Aligners

Today, plastic aligners are a mainstay of orthodontic treatment. Clinicians are now able to truly design the smile in real time and to deliver optimum orthodontic results in a predictable manner. Once the teeth have been scanned by an intraoral scanner, the teeth may be visualized in 3 dimensions and carefully manipulated to achieve the

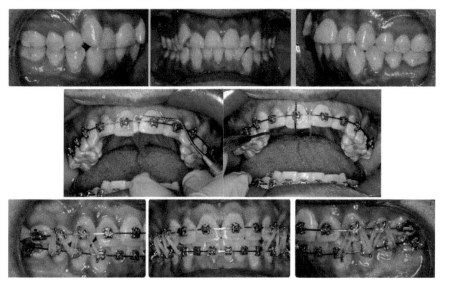

Fig. 7. Careful buildup and selective IPR of the anterior zone of teeth by the author (C.H.K.). This simple and effective process helps to guide the clinician in the management of the smile zone and careful smile design of the individual patient.

desired occlusion. This visual map of teeth can also help the patient gain the idea of what to expect. Modifications/customizations of tooth size, tooth movement, and final positions can be made unique to each tooth. Diagnosis and treatment planning for a pleasing smile is made easy through 3D visualization. Mock treatment plans help the orthodontist to make decisions and experiment with various treatment plans without actually delivering the appliances to the patient (**Figs. 8** and **9**). Once the desired treatment plan is agreed upon, the aligners are fabricated by the companies and shipped to the orthodontic practices or sometimes directly to patient. In the subsequent visits to the clinic, orthodontist carefully monitors the progression of plastic aligner therapy and each aligner is worn for 20 to 22 hours per day for up to 10 days. The tight fit of the aligner around each allows the plastic to place the desired pressure on the biological system remodeling bone and creating the desired tooth movements. When more complex tooth movements are required, clear composite tooth material is placed to act as an attachment so that the plastic aligners can have a better "grip" to bring about tooth movement.

Peg Lateral or Missing Lateral: Buildup or Canine Substitution

The treatment of patients with missing lateral incisors is often a multidisciplinary dental specialty approach; it involves orthodontics, esthetic dentistry, implantology, and prosthodontics. The team approach ensures that an optimal occlusion along with a well-balanced stable natural smile is achieved.

In the anterior smiling zone, there are various treatment options. In fact, there are 3 different options to manage the missing lateral incisors. These options include canine substitution, a tooth-supported restoration, and a single tooth implant. All options

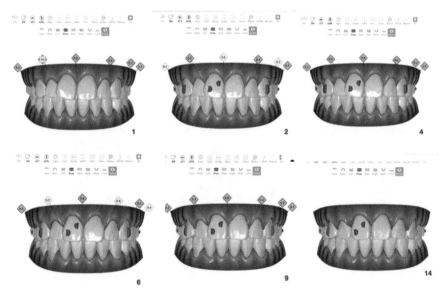

Fig. 8. An example of a computer-generated representation of tooth movements. The dentition was captured by the iTero intraoral scanner (Align Technology, San Jose, California) and uploaded as a stereolithography model into the aligner software (Smartee Systems, Shanghai, China). A total of 14 aligners were required to bring about tooth movement and tooth alignment. IPR and composite attachments are also prescribed during treatment sequence.

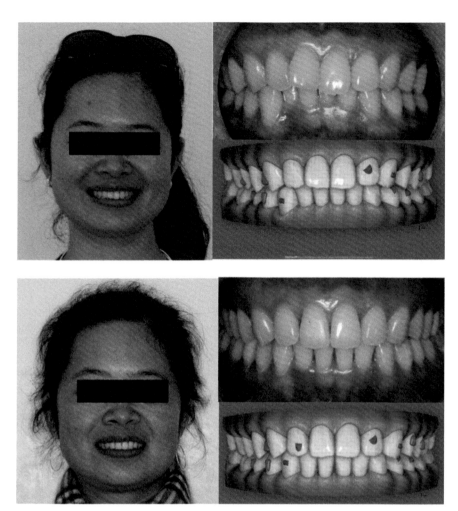

Fig. 9. Smile design using Invisalign software (Align Technology, San Jose, CA, USA). The initial and final 3D rendering are seen together with the before and after smiles of the patient. The effective delivery of the treatment plan with plastic aligners has made these aligner systems popular among patients.

should be thoroughly discussed with the patient and/or parents, and the advantages and disadvantages of each treatment option should be explained.[47–49] The main objective of treatment planning should be tooth conservation wherein the least invasive option that satisfies the expected esthetic and functional objectives is prescribed.[50] Various factors should be considered by an orthodontist while treatment planning. We discuss the canine substitution and tooth-supported restoration for the treatment of missing lateral incisors.

Canine substitution
The most appropriate patient for this procedure has an Angle class II malocclusion with no crowding in the mandibular arch, has a class II molar relationship with canines in traditional position, or has Angle class I malocclusion with sufficient crowding to necessitate mandibular extractions. By substituting the canines, the final result will

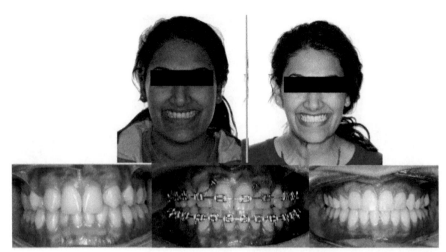

Fig. 10. Canine substitution with anterior TAD support (Ormco VectroTAS System, Drea, CA, USA).

require the premolars take the load of the chewing cycle, and therefore the resulting occlusal scheme should be "group" function. As orthodontists the shape and color of the canine are also important esthetic factors for consideration. While reducing the canine to re-create normal lateral contours, clinicians also need to prevent of dentine or pulpal exposure.

To correct the color difference, bleaching the canine may be done failing which a veneer can be placed. The crown width at the CEJ should be evaluated on a pretreatment radiograph to help determine the final emergence profile, and the gingival margin of the natural canine should be positioned slightly incisal to the central incisor gingival margin. Simple gingivectomies described previously can also be done to achieve this. Proper bracket placement is important too if regular braces are used. Each bracket should be placed according to the gingival margin height rather than incisal edge or cusp tip. After the teeth have been aligned, restorative treatment may be needed to re-create an ideal lateral incisor color and contour. If these steps are followed, satisfactory esthetic outcomes can be achieved without causing functional problems to arise within the temporomandibular joint and allows periodontal health conditions to be better maintained (**Fig. 10**).

Tooth-supported restoration
When the goal is to restore the missing or small teeth, tooth-supported restorations are considered. The primary types of tooth-supported restorations are resin-bonded fixed partial denture, a cantilevered-fixed partial denture, and a conventional full coverage fixed partial denture. The main objective while treating a peg-shaped lateral by the restorative treatment options should be tooth conservation, to achieve predictable esthetics, function, and longevity.[40] Again, the planning and execution involves a multidisciplinary approach to treat such cases. Thorough discussion of the case of missing maxillary lateral incisor or the presence of a peg-shaped lateral incisor should be done by an orthodontist with a restorative dentist before starting the treatment.[48]

The orthodontist plays an important role to determine and establish space requirements for patients with missing maxillary lateral incisor. The various methods to

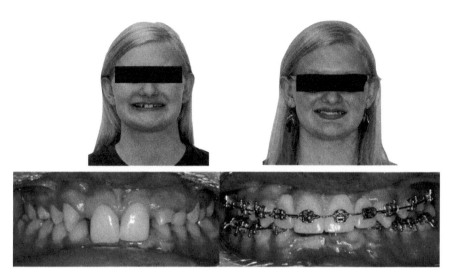

Fig. 11. Lateral incisors buildup using denture teeth attached to orthodontic archwires. The plastic pontic teeth are attached to regular orthodontic brackets and mounted onto a regular archwire. Ligature tie wires are used to secure the brackets and prevent unwanted movement of teeth.

determine this are the golden proportion, using the contralateral lateral incisor as a guide, or to conduct a Bolton analysis. In some cases in which there is a bilateral involvement of 2 missing lateral incisors, the use of denture pontic teeth can be extremely useful (**Fig. 11**). In complex cases, a diagnostic wax up is the most predictable guide for determining ideal space.[48]

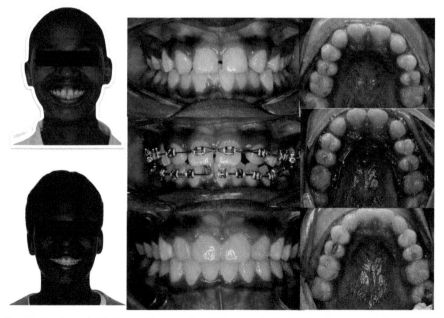

Fig. 12. Canine substitution with posterior TAD support. The TAD system used is the BENEFIT System (PSM Medical Solutions, Gunnigen, Germany) developed by Dr Benedict Wilmes.[53]

Control of Torque for Facial Balance: Protraction with Temporary Anchorage Devicesor Retraction with Temporary Anchorage Devices

The application of temporary anchorage devices (TADs) is well known for its effectiveness in the intrusion, extrusion, protraction, and retraction of the anterior or posterior teeth.[51] Orthodontists mostly plan treatment involving closing or opening of spaces. Sometimes to do so, some form of rigid anchor is required, and TADs have become increasing popular and are often indicated.[47–49]

TADs allow movement of teeth that require heavy anchorage with the orthodontic biomechanical system. If TADs are placed posterior and bilaterally on each side, this ensures the line of action of force passes through the center of resistance of the anterior teeth; this allows teeth intrusion or distal movement of teeth.[52] TADs placed in the interdental bone between the maxillary first molar and second premolar prove to be efficient for intraoral anchorage reinforcements for en masse retraction and intrusion of the maxillary anterior teeth. The vertical position of the TADs plays a characterizing job in coordinating the forces applied in intruding and extruding the anterior teeth. The forces did not gather at a single point and were distributed in root areas of teeth because of the group movement of teeth. This, along with the way that spaces distal to the lateral incisors that are obvious after individual canine retraction never show up with en masse retraction incredibly upgrades patient collaboration and inspiration. The TADs are put in the interdental bone between the maxillary first molar and second premolar and end up being productive for intraoral anchorage fortifications for en masse retraction and intrusion of the maxillary front teeth. In some instances, TADs may also be placed in the palate and hence do interfere with tooth movement within the arch (**Fig. 12**).

SUMMARY

Orthodontists play a vital role in the smile design of individuals. There are a variety of orthodontic goals and tooth movements that can be achieved to obtain the ideal smile that ultimately leads to the optimum esthetic outcomes. In this article, some methods and appliance systems to control and achieve the desired tooth movements are described and illustrated.

DISCLOSURE

The authors do not have financial or commercial conflicts of interest when writing this article. The authors have not used any funding source or grant agency in the preparation of the manuscript.

REFERENCES

1. Christou T, Betlej A, Aswad N, et al. Clinical effectiveness of orthodontic treatment on smile esthetics: a systematic review. Clin Cosmet Investig Dent 2019;11: 89–101.
2. Hulsey CM. An esthetic evaluation of lip-teeth relationships present in the smile. Am J Orthod 1970;57(2):132–44.
3. Christou T, Abarca R, Christou V, et al. Smile outcome comparison of Invisalign and traditional fixed-appliance treatment: A case-control study. Am J Orthod Dentofacial Orthop 2020;157(3):357–64.
4. Sarver DM. The importance of incisor positioning in the esthetic smile: the smile arc. Am J Orthod Dentofacial Orthop 2001;120(2):98–111.

5. Ackerman MB, Ackerman JL. Smile analysis and design in the digital era. J Clin Orthod 2002;36(4):221–36.
6. Kau CH, Christou T, Xie RB, et al. Rating of smile attractiveness of patients finished to the American Board of Orthodontics standards. J Orofac Orthop 2020;81(4):239–48.
7. Soh J, Wang ZD, Zhang WB, et al. Smile attractiveness evaluation of patients selected for a u.s.-based board certification examination. Eur J Dent 2021; 15(4):630–8.
8. Krishnan V, Daniel ST, Lazar D, et al. Characterization of posed smile by using visual analog scale, smile arc, buccal corridor measures, and modified smile index. Am J Orthod Dentofacial Orthop 2008;133(4):515–23.
9. Cheng HC, Wang YC, Tam KW, et al. Effects of tooth extraction on smile esthetics and the buccal corridor: A meta-analysis. J Dent Sci 2016;11(4):387–93.
10. Kokich VO Jr, Kiyak HA, Shapiro PA. Comparing the perception of dentists and lay people to altered dental esthetics. J Esthet Dent 1999;11(6):311–24.
11. Sarver D. Smile projection-a new concept in smile design. J Esthet Restor Dent 2021;33(1):237–52.
12. Machado AW, Moon W, Gandini LG Jr. Influence of maxillary incisor edge asymmetries on the perception of smile esthetics among orthodontists and laypersons. Am J Orthod Dentofacial Orthop 2013;143(5):658–64.
13. Machado AW, McComb RW, Moon W, et al. Influence of the vertical position of maxillary central incisors on the perception of smile esthetics among orthodontists and laypersons. J Esthet Restor Dent 2013;25(6):392–401.
14. Machado AW. 10 commandments of smile esthetics. Dental Press J Orthod 2014; 19(4):136–57.
15. Wolfart S, Thormann H, Freitag S, et al. Assessment of dental appearance following changes in incisor proportions. Eur J Oral Sci 2005;113(2):159–65.
16. Kokich VO, Kokich VG, Kiyak HA. Perceptions of dental professionals and laypersons to altered dental esthetics: asymmetric and symmetric situations. Am J Orthod Dentofacial Orthop 2006;130(2):141–51.
17. Sadowsky SJ. An overview of treatment considerations for esthetic restorations: a review of the literature. J Prosthet Dent 2006;96(6):433–42.
18. Dunn WJ, Murchison DF, Broome JC. Esthetics: patients' perceptions of dental attractiveness. J Prosthodont 1996;5(3):166–71.
19. Heravi F, Rashed R, Abachizadeh H. Esthetic preferences for the shape of anterior teeth in a posed smile. Am J Orthod Dentofacial Orthop 2011;139(6):806–14.
20. Ong E, Brown RA, Richmond S. Peer assessment of dental attractiveness. Am J Orthod Dentofacial Orthop 2006;130(2):163–9.
21. Lombardi RE. The principles of visual perception and their clinical application to denture esthetics. The J Prosthetic Dentistry 1973;29(4):358–82.
22. Ward DH. A study of dentists' preferred maxillary anterior tooth width proportions: comparing the recurring esthetic dental proportion to other mathematical and naturally occurring proportions. J Esthet Restor Dent 2007;19(6):324–37, discussion 38-9.
23. Frush JP, Fisher RD. The dynesthetic interpretation of the dentogenic concept. J Prosthetic Dentistry 1958;8(4):558–81.
24. Bhuvaneswaran M. Principles of smile design. J Conserv Dent 2010;13(4): 225–32.
25. Sabri R. The eight components of a balanced smile. J Clin Orthod 2005;39(3): 155–67, quiz 54.

26. McNamara L, McNamara JA Jr, Ackerman MB, et al. Hard- and soft-tissue contributions to the esthetics of the posed smile in growing patients seeking orthodontic treatment. Am J Orthod Dentofacial Orthop 2008;133(4):491–9.

27. Torassian G, Kau CH, English JD, et al. Digital models vs plaster models using alginate and alginate substitute materials. Angle Orthod 2010;80(4):474–81.

28. Pan F, Kau CH, Zhou H, et al. The anatomical evaluation of the dental arches using cone beam computed tomography–an investigation of the availability of bone for placement of mini-screws. Head Face Med 2013;9:13.

29. O'Neil R, Kau CH. Comparison of dental arch forms created from assessment of teeth, alveolar bone, and the overlying soft tissue. J Orofac Orthop 2021;82(6): 413–21.

30. Gor T, Kau CH, English JD, et al. Three-dimensional comparison of facial morphology in white populations in Budapest, Hungary, and Houston, Texas. Am J Orthod Dentofacial Orthop 2010;137(3):424–32.

31. Kau CH. Creation of the virtual patient for the study of facial morphology. Facial Plast Surg Clin North Am 2011;19(4):615–22, viii.

32. Wong ME, Kau CH, Melville JC, et al. Bone reconstruction planning using computer technology for surgical management of severe maxillomandibular atrophy. Oral Maxillofac Surg Clin North Am 2019;31(3):457–72.

33. Kau CH, Wang Z, Wang J, et al. Contemporary management of an orthodontic-orthognathic patient with limited time availability in an orthodontic office setting: case report. J Orthod 2020. 1465312520934488.

34. Kyteas PG, McKenzie WS, Waite PD, et al. Comprehensive treatment approach for condylar hyperplasia and mandibular crowding with custom lingual braces and 2-jaw surgery. Am J Orthod Dentofacial Orthop 2017;151(1):174–85.

35. Veiszenbacher E, Wang J, Davis M, et al. Virtual surgical planning: balancing esthetics, practicality, and anticipated stability in a complex Class III patient. Am J Orthod Dentofacial Orthop 2019;156(5):685–93.

36. Aslanidou K, Xie R, Christou T, et al. Evaluation of temporomandibular joint function after orthognathic surgery using a jaw tracker. J Orthod 2020. 1465312520908277.

37. He S, Kau CH, Liao L, et al. The use of a dynamic real-time jaw tracking device and cone beam computed tomography simulation. Ann Maxillofac Surg 2016; 6(1):113–9.

38. Mercado-Garcia J, Rosso P, Gonzalvez-Garcia M, et al. Gummy smile: mercado-rosso classification system and dynamic restructuring with hyaluronic acid. Aesthet Plast Surg 2021.

39. Mohamed Ali J, Ines D. Orthodontics gummy smile. Treasure Island (FL): StatPearls; 2021.

40. Oueis R, Waite PD, Wang J, et al. Orthodontic-Orthognathic Management of a patient with skeletal class II with bimaxillary protrusion, complicated by vertical maxillary excess: a multi-faceted case report of difficult treatment management issues. Int Orthod 2020;18(1):178–90.

41. Polo M. Botulinum toxin type a (botox) for the neuromuscular correction of excessive gingival display on smiling (gummy smile). Am J Orthod Dentofacial Orthop 2008;133(2):195–203.

42. Silberberg N, Goldstein M, Smidt A. Excessive gingival display–etiology, diagnosis, and treatment modalities. Quintessence Int 2009;40(10):809–18.

43. Coslet JG, Vanarsdall R, Weisgold A. Diagnosis and classification of delayed passive eruption of the dentogingival junction in the adult. Alpha Omegan 1977;70(3):24–8.

44. Li JL, Kau C, Wang M. Changes of occlusal plane inclination after orthodontic treatment in different dentoskeletal frames. Prog Orthod 2014;15(1):41.

45. Pitts TR. Bracket positioning for smile arc protection. J Clin Orthod 2017;51(3): 142–56.

46. Kau CH, Bakos K, Lamani E. Quantifying changes in incisor inclination before and after orthodontic treatment in class I, II, and III malocclusions. J World Fed Orthod 2020;9(4):170–4.

47. Kokich VO Jr, Kinzer GA. Managing congenitally missing lateral incisors. part I: canine substitution. J Esthet Restor Dent 2005;17(1):5–10.

48. Kinzer GA, Kokich VO Jr. Managing congenitally missing lateral incisors. part II: tooth-supported restorations. J Esthet Restor Dent 2005;17(2):76–84.

49. Kinzer GA, Kokich VO Jr. Managing congenitally missing lateral incisors. part III: single-tooth implants. J Esthet Restor Dent 2005;17(4):202–10.

50. Holm U. [Problems of the closing of spaces and compensatory extraction in agenesis of upper lateral incisors]. Fortschr Kieferorthop 1971;32(2):233–47.

51. Kau CH, Christou T. TADs and Successful Clinical Outcomes. In: Park JH, editor. Temporary anchorage devices in clinical orthodontics. Hoboken (NJ): Wiley-Blackwell; 2020. p. 69–76.

52. Baek ES, Hwang S, Kim KH, et al. Total intrusion and distalization of the maxillary arch to improve smile esthetics. Korean J Orthod 2017;47(1):59–73.

53. Wilmes B, Nienkemper M, Ludwig B, et al. Esthetic Class II treatment with the Beneslider and aligners. J Clin Orthod 2012;46(7):390–8, quiz 437.

Smile Design
Mechanical Considerations

Marzieh Alikhasi, DDS, MS[a],*, Parisa Yousefi, DDS, MS[b],
Kelvin I. Afrashtehfar, DDS, MSc, Dr med dent, FDS RCSEng, FRCD(C)[c,d],*

KEYWORDS

- Artificial intelligence • Augmented reality • Dentures • Digital technology • Esthetics
- Patient satisfaction • Prosthodontics

KEY POINTS

- Adherence to the primary reconstruction principles permits achieving durable esthetic outcomes.
- Dental clinicians should provide a realistic image of the expected esthetic outcomes to their patients.
- The use of digital treatment planning tools does not undermine the significance of the prosthodontic concepts that were born during the fully conventional era.

INTRODUCTION

A smile is a facial expression of emotions through the contraction of facial expression muscles to display the maxillary teeth, which can commonly influence how an individual fits and functions in society.[1] The lips act as the smile framework exposing teeth referred to as the esthetic zone.[2,3] Smile designing refers to the cosmetic and esthetic teeth reconstruction that is primarily displayed during smiling. Esthetic dentistry is not a separate discipline or field of dentistry[4]; instead, it is the ultimate goal of most therapeutic interventions and procedures performed in different dental specialties.[5,6] In the recent years, dental interventions seem to be more frequently becoming appearance-driven, and thus, both patients and dental clinicians mainly emphasize on esthetic dental and facial aspects of treatments. Consequently, reconstructive

[a] Dental Implant Research Center, Dentistry Research Institute, Tehran University of Medical Sciences, Tehran 1439955991, Iran; [b] Department of Prosthodontics, School of Dentistry, Isfahan University of Medical Sciences, Hezar Jarib Street, Isfahan 8174673461, Isfahan Province, Iran; [c] Evidence-Based Practice Unit, Disciplines of Prosthodontology and Implantology, Division of Restorative Dental Sciences, Clinical Sciences Department, Ajman University College of Dentistry, PO Box 346 Ajman City, Ajman Emirate, UAE; [d] Department of Reconstructive Dentistry & Gerodontology, School of Dental Medicine (ZMK), Faculty of Medicine, University of Bern, Freiburgstrasse 7, Bern 3010, BE, Switzerland
* Corresponding authors.
E-mail addresses: malikhasi@razi.tums.ac.ir (M.A.); kelvin.afrashtehfar@zmk.unibe.ch (K.I.A.)

Dent Clin N Am 66 (2022) 477–487
https://doi.org/10.1016/j.cden.2022.02.008
0011-8532/22/© 2022 The Author(s). Published by Elsevier Inc. This is an open access article under the CC BY-NC-ND license (http://creativecommons.org/licenses/by-nc-nd/4.0/).
dental.theclinics.com

dentistry pursues objectives beyond the reconstruction of severely carious or damaged teeth.

Misconceptions About Reconstructive Dental Procedures to Enhance the Appearance

Increasing people's awareness regarding the importance and impact of healthy teeth and beautiful smile on various aspects of life such as social acceptance and self-confidence,[7,8] and frequent exposure to patterns advertised as a measure of beauty in social networks has increased the demand for a smile makeover procedures.[9,10] When patient awareness is minimal or distorted, their altered perceptions could persuade them to demand results that do not mimic nature. For instance, patients' perception of an ideal smile could correspond to having super white and oversized teeth.[11] However, patients should also be well aware of such treatments' consequences, risks, and limitations of such treatments. For example, ceramic veneers that reportedly require no tooth preparation have received significant publicity and continue to being available by various trade names. As a result, many patients that seek a smile enhancement procedure believe that optimal smile esthetics can be achieved only by "prepless" veneers. Although tooth structure preservation is a priority, some cases require a less conservative approach as 0.3 mm thick ceramic veneer can reduce one tone (eg, A3 to A2). Masking of an achromatic abutment requires more aggressive preparations to modify several shade tones.[12] Besides, it is well established that ceramic veneers bonded to enamel have high survival and retrievability of sound enamel even with no-prep veneers is not possible.[13,14] It is fundamental to realize that each case is different, and one solution does not fit all. This appeals to the personalized medicine concept.

Dental clinicians and technicians achieve ideal esthetic results in prosthodontics when performing a correct individualized diagnosis, planning, and execution considering the tooth position, tooth preparation design, contour and color of restoration and stump, and material selection. Also, preprosthetic corrective orthodontics may be an adjunct to upright a mesially tilted molar or improve the teeth' position within the arch or occlusion to offer less aggressive prosthetic preparations and favor the longevity and prognosis of the overall prognosis treatment.[15–17] In other cases, preprosthetic surgical alterations such as recontouring of gingival margin may be required to achieve favorable esthetic results.[18]

Prosthodontic Digital Diagnostic Aids

Digital technology can be used to visually predict the esthetic treatment outcome and present it to patients, increasing the patient treatment acceptance rate. Many of these software programs are based on the concept of digital smile design (DSD) approach introduced by Ackermann[19] and Coachman.[20] Objective transfer of such computer-aided designs (CADs) from the software applications such as Adobe Photoshop, PowerPoint, and Keynote to the oral environment is not always feasible. Some newer generations of such programs enable three-dimensional (3D) and even four-dimensional designs (simulating movements) to overcome many of the abovementioned limitations.[21,22] However, it should be noted that this virtual smile proposal could sometimes be unrealistic and unachievable due to the skeletal relations, occlusion, and dental arch form are overlooked. Nonetheless, the use of novel advanced digital tools does not undermine the significance of adherence to the main prosthodontic principles. The creation of a pleasing smile requires simultaneous consideration of psychological, biological, and mechanical factors. Introduction of esthetic wheel and defining esthetic dimensions are attempts to find the influential factors involved in the creating of an attractive smile.[23,24] The mechanical features that are integrated into prosthodontic treatment are further discussed.

MECHANICAL FACTORS

Mechanical factors may be considered as the cornerstone of reconstructive dentistry. **Fig. 1** denotes the 4 aspects of a tooth that should be considered when restoring a natural maxillary tooth, dental implant, or even using a denture tooth in the esthetic zone. Generally, patients and some dental clinicians only focus on the labial/buccal and incisal aspects to achieve dental esthetics and neglect the cervical (emergence profile) and lingual aspects. The 4 aspects should be correctly addressed in reconstructions to achieve optimal long-term esthetic and functional outcomes respecting biological factors.

Incisal Edge

Patients' expectations from dental reconstructions in the esthetic zone often depend on the incisal edge's location and form. Patients usually demand longer incisors than their existing teeth. Different optimal mean and rage values of incisal edge show at rest have been proposed according to the age and sex of the patient. Most often, 2 to 4 mm of incisal edge show is preferred at rest. The entire cervico-incisal length of the anterior maxillary teeth should be preferably visible when smiling. The width/height ratio and the height/face ratio are among the indices used to calculate the ideal amount of tooth show. It appears that the final value should better be determined based on the individual preferences and conditions of each patient.[8,25,26] First, the

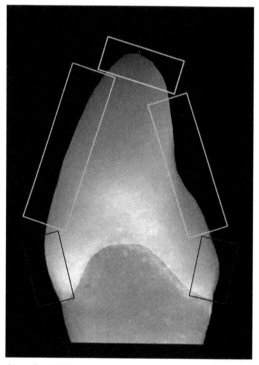

Fig. 1. Incisal (*green*), occlusal (*blue*), labial (*yellow*), and cervical (*red*) parts of a tooth or implant should be considered for reconstruction.

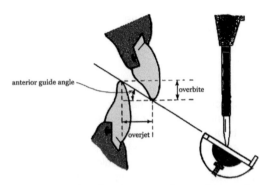

Fig. 2. Increasing the crown height often increases the overbite and anterior guidance.

amount of incisal edge display of the 2 central incisors is determined, and then the presumed value is tried in. We can use these methods for the primary assessment of the presumed values:

- Clinically designed mock-up: The clinician generates a mock-up in the patient's mouth with incremental composite resin without acid-etching or adhesive
- Conventional laboratory designed mock-up: A diagnostic wax-up is transferred to the patient's mouth via a silicone index
- Use of two-dimensional designing software programs
- Use of exclusive 3D DSD software programs

When DSD software programs are used, the required photographs are obtained, the incisal edge location and the amount of incisal display are determined as the starting point. In the conventional workflow, a diagnostic wax-up should be first done. For diagnostic waxing, technicians often calculate the correct length/width ratio of central incisors (70%–85%) as the starting point.[27] Thus, in most cases, the crown height obtained by digital mock-up design is often different from that obtained by diagnostic wax-up on a cast.[28] Photographs or videos can be obtained to guide technicians for conventional laboratory waxing. Restorative dentists should assess whether increasing the crown height is feasible within the prosthodontic parameters below mentioned:

- Crown/root ratio
- Anterior guidance
- Posterior disclusion
- Phonetics
- Envelope of motion

A patient that undergoes a crown lengthening that includes osteotomy for leveling of the gingival margin and zenith loses part of the bone support. Increasing the crown height for esthetic purposes can further aggravate the situation because the increased crown/root ratio can affect the longevity and survival of the respective tooth. Moreover, increasing the crown height alters the overbite and anterior guidance (**Fig. 2**). Although achieving a mutually protected occlusion is optional, the magnitude of posterior teeth disclusion due to the mandibular excursions should be within normal limits (range: 1–4 mm).[29] Higher values promote lateral forces with unfavorable direction and detrimental magnitude on anterior teeth.[30] Furthermore, if not accompanied by increased overjet (infrequently feasible), increased overbite can limit the envelope of function (**Fig. 3**), and lead to patient discomfort and dissatisfaction.[31]

In addition to the incisal edge position, the incisal plane is a critical factor. In the conventional workflow, a face-bow transfers the current incisal slope relative to the horizontal plane to the articulator. Reference horizontal plane is parallel to the pupils or, in case of facial asymmetry, parallel to the correct horizontal plane of the patient's face to the laboratory. In the digital workflow, this transfer is performed by drawing the respective lines on the face and teeth.[32] To determine the incisal plane, the lower lip curvature (smile line) can be used in software programs. In the conventional workflow, this line can be somewhat drawn on the cast. A consonant smile can be achieved when an imaginary line running from the incisal edges of the maxillary incisors follows the smile line curvature correctly.

Labial Surface

The labial surface is the second determining factor that affects dental esthetics. Mesiodistal width is one of the parameters that should be considered to form the labial surface correctly. The golden ratio has long been used to achieve optimal symmetry, dominance, and dental proportions in the anterior maxillary teeth.[33] Different criteria have been proposed to determine the mesiodistal dimensions of teeth, such as the recurring esthetic dental proportion, golden proportion, facial analysis, and repeated ratio.[34–36] In the digital workflow, proportion tools are used to determine these proportions. However, these ideal proportions cannot be achieved in all cases. Factors that interfere with achieving ideal tooth width proportions include:

- Interdental spaces
- Crowding
- Microdontia

The labial surface convexity also affects the visible width of teeth. The buccal corridor must be minimal in an ideal smile but should not be eliminated (**Fig. 4**A and

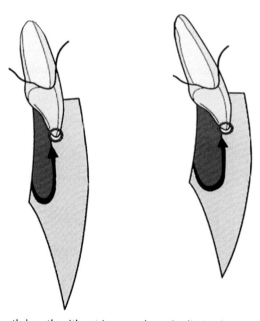

Fig. 3. Changing tooth length without increased overjet limits the envelope of function.

B).[37–39] When a tooth dimension is determined, the outline should be defined, which refers to designing the tooth shape based on the patient's personality, facial form, and preferences.[8,26] The technician manually generates a conventional wax-up by taking all factors into account, whereas in the digital workflow, this process is supported by CAD software programs. The dental outline is determined using software programs teeth libraries. Designing software programs facilitate this process such that even novice dental clinicians may have difficulties molding the tooth shape directly with composite resins or indirectly on wax to achieve a correct tooth form and shape. However, an experienced operator who digitally designs by CAD can create an acceptable smile in a shorter time.[40]

Occlusal Surface

A comfortable and stable occlusion is the key to a long-term successful prosthetic treatment. Centric occlusion, centric relation, vertical dimension of occlusion, and eccentric movements are among the primary parameters to consider when restoring occlusal parts. Occlusion is less commonly affected in cases whereby only the labial surface is veneered without an incisal overlap design (ie, window preparation). In such cases, the only occlusal modification is related to the incisal edge height. Nonetheless, many patients that seek esthetic dental reconstructions require alterations of the occlusal surface due to the following specific conditions:

- Tooth wear (attrition, erosion)
- Requiring an increase in vertical height
- Jaw mal-relationship
- Dental caries
- Structural damage (fractures, craze lines)

Occlusal aspects may be neglected in esthetic treatments, leading to unpredictable and unstable treatment outcomes. Despite the primary concepts regarding the inability to increase the vertical occlusal height, stable results may be achieved if it is performed correctly.[14] Correct occlusal management and equilibration require ample knowledge and adequate expertise in the field. Some noteworthy key points in this respect include:

- The envelope of function should not be limited as the patient feels that teeth are trapped or locked in a limited area (see **Fig. 3**).[41]

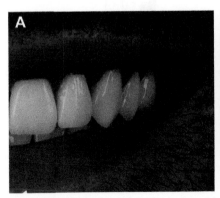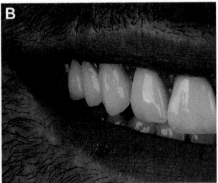

Fig. 4. (*A*) Acceptable uniform buccal corridor. (*B*) The corridor is not uniform and is prominent in the molar area.

- A mutually protected occlusion should be achieved.
- Reconstruction should be performed with normal disclusion of posterior teeth in eccentric movements.
- The concavity of the cingulum area should be correctly designed to allow freedom in centric and correct guidance[42] (**Fig. 5**A and B).

The interim restoration is a blueprint of the future definitive reconstruction while being easily modified while assessing all these parameters. CAD files do not substitute interim restorations because the prototype shall be tested intraorally even if the patient accepts the 2D design. CAD/computer-aided manufacturing technology (CAM) has been used to fabricate interim restorations, and temporary materials used for milling or printing are more homogenous than direct temporary composites or acrylic materials.[43]

Cervical Region

The cervical region of the teeth is both esthetically and biologically important due to the proximity to the gingival margin. As mentioned earlier, the entire crown height and even part of the gingiva may be visible in a beautiful smile. The cervical tooth contour and periodontal health play a pivotal role in the treatment outcome. Dental restorations, once considered as "cosmetic solutions," should be removed when causing significant inflammation to the adjacent gingiva. Thus, concepts such as emergence profile and axial contours, as well as supracrestal attachment (formerly known as biologic width), should emulate nature and avoid overcontoured restorations or invading soft tissues. The cervical region analysis includes the assessment of gingival morphology, interdental papilla condition, gingival zenith position, gingival line, and gingival contour.

PSYCHOLOGICAL FACTORS

People try to cover their mouth or hide their teeth when they are dissatisfied with their smile appearance. This could be seen when a subject presents misalignment, discoloration, staining, or missing teeth. Investigations have revealed that having an attractive smile is directly linked to higher self-confidence and satisfaction.[1,3,44] A clinician is required to evaluate the patient's chief complaints by thoroughly analyzing the patient's mental state before designing a treatment plan.[45] The potential of artificial intelligence (AI) and virtual reality/augmented reality (VR/AR) technologies are solutions that rapidly evolved and can help patients and clinicians visualize treatment outcomes

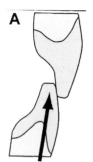 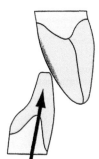 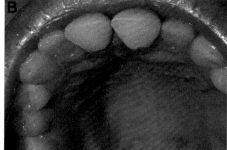

Fig. 5. (*A*) The anatomic contour does not follow a concave outline and lacks a stable contact. (*B*) Convex cingulum area increases traumatic forces on the tooth.

before any clinical intervention.[46–51] The goal is to have the clinician's treatment plan and the patient's demands as close to each other as possible. In many cases, the reason for patients' dissatisfaction with their smile appearance does not depend on technical issues. These are situations in which patients need serious psychological counseling to become aware of the true nature of their problem.[52,53]

BIOLOGICAL FACTORS

The condition of several intraoral and extraoral elements such as the periodontium complex, perioral muscles, skeletal components of the jaws, and how the expression of a smile communicates with adjacent components, including the nose and chin, all have undeniable effects on the beauty of a smile. Therefore, all specialists involved in the treatment should confirm the smile design. In most cases, the ideal status of the factors mentioned is a serious precondition for achieving an ideal outcome in smile design.

SUMMARY

As long as the demand for enhancing teeth appearance increases, restorative materials and technologies will continue developing to meet society's needs. The main advances have occurred in bleaching techniques, dental restorative materials, smile designing programs, prosthetic techniques, and bonding agents. The incorporation of digital 3D designing into AI and machine learning has also contributed to this process. The use of modern digital tools requires adequate knowledge about the tooth form and shape principles that have been sufficiently revised and documented. The mechanical, biological, and psychological factors should not be overlooked to achieve favorable esthetics. The durability of an esthetic restoration depends on adherence to the established principles of reconstruction.

CONFLICT OF INTEREST AND SOURCE OF FUNDING

The authors do not have any financial interests, either directly or indirectly, in the products or information enclosed in the article.

CLINICS CARE POINTS

- The creation of a pleasing smile requires simultaneous consideration of psychological, biological, and mechanical factors.
- If not accompanied by increased overjet, increased overbite can limit the envelope of function, and lead to patient discomfort and dissatisfaction.
- Reconstruction should be performed with normal disclusion of posterior teeth in eccentric movements.
- Concepts such as emergence profile and axial contours, as well as supracrestal attachment should emulate nature and avoid overcontoured restorations or invading soft tissues.

REFERENCES

1. Beall AE. Can a new smile make you look more intelligent and successful? Dent Clin North Am 2007;51(2):289–97.

2. Salama H, Salama M, Garber D, et al. Developing optimal peri-implant papillae within the esthetic zone: guided soft tissue augmentation. J Esthet Restor Dent 1995;7(3):125–9.

3. Afrashtehfar KI, Assery MK, Bryant SR. Aesthetic parameters and patient-perspective assessment tools for maxillary anterior single implants. Int J Dent 2021;2021.

4. Heymann HO, Paravina RD, Blatz MB. Advances in esthetic dentistry 2021. J Esthet Restor Dent 2021;33(1):5–6.

5. Touyz LZ, Raviv E, Harel-Raviv M. Cosmetic or esthetic dentistry? Quintessence Int 1999;30(4).

6. Goldstein RE. Study of need for esthetics in dentistry. J Prosthet Dent 1969;21(6): 589–98.

7. Van der Geld P, Oosterveld P, Van Heck G, et al. Smile attractiveness: self-perception and influence on personality. Angle Orthod 2007;77(5):759–65.

8. Del Monte S, Afrashtehfar KI, Emami E, et al. Lay preferences for dentogingival esthetic parameters: a systematic review. J Prosthet Dent 2017;118(6):717–24.

9. Wooi M. Smile makeover generation? Br Dent J 2021;230(7):387.

10. Dorfman WM. A real-life hollywood success story: how extreme makeovers can make you a star. J Indiana Dent Assoc 2006;85(1):8–12.

11. Magne P, Salem P, Magne M. Influence of symmetry and balance on visual perception of a white female smile. J Prosthet Dent 2018;120(4):573–82.

12. Coachman C, Gurel G, Calamita M, et al. The influence of tooth color on preparation design for laminate veneers from a minimally invasive perspective: case report. Int J Periodontics Restorative Dent 2014;34(4).

13. Gurel G, Sesma N, Calamita MA, et al. Influence of enamel preservation on failure rates of porcelain laminate veneers. Int J Periodontics Restorative Dent 2013;33(1).

14. Layton DM, Clarke M. A systematic review and meta-analysis of the survival of non-feldspathic porcelain veneers over 5 and 10 years. Int J Prosthodont 2013;26(2).

15. Bidra AS, Uribe F. Preprosthetic orthodontic intervention for management of a partially edentulous patient with generalized wear and malocclusion. J Esthet Restor Dent 2012;24(2):88–100.

16. Wiskott A, Schatz J, Belser U. Preprosthetic orthodontics. 1. theoretical bases. Schweiz Monatsschr Zahnmed 1988;98(4):372–82.

17. Alfallaj H. Pre-prosthetic orthodontics. Saudi Dent J 2020;32(1):7–14.

18. Nemcovsky C, Artzi Z, Moses O. Preprosthetic clinical crown lengthening procedures in the anterior maxilla. Practical procedures & aesthetic dentistry. Pract Proced Aesthet Dent 2001;13(7):581–8, quiz 9.

19. Ackerman MB, Ackerman JL. Smile analysis and design in the digital era. J Clin Orthod 2002;36(4):221–36.

20. Coachman C, Paravina RD. Digitally enhanced esthetic dentistry-From treatment planning to quality control. J Esthet Restor Dent, 28 (Suppl 1), 2016, S3-4.

21. Marchand L, Touati R, Fehmer V, et al. Latest advances in augmented reality technology and its integration into the digital workflow. Int J Comput Dent 2020;23(4): 397–408.

22. Kurbad A. The use of 'extended reality'(augmented reality) in esthetic treatment planning Der Einsatz der "erweiterten Realität "(Augmented Reality) in der ästhetischen Planung. Int J Comput Dent 2020;23(2):149–60.

23. Gürel G. The fifth dimension in esthetic dentistry. Bulgaria: University of Sofia; 2021.

24. Koirala S. Smile design wheel™: a practical approach to smile design. Cosmet dentistry 2009;3(3):24–8.

25. Witt M, Flores-Mir C. Laypeople's preferences regarding frontal dentofacial esthetics: periodontal factors. J Am Dent Assoc 2011;142(8):925–37.

26. Parrini S, Rossini G, Castroflorio T, et al. Laypeople's perceptions of frontal smile esthetics: A systematic review. Am J Orthod Dentofacial Orthop 2016;150(5): 740–50.

27. Blatz M, Chiche G, Bahat O, et al. Evolution of aesthetic dentistry. J Dent Res 2019;98(12):1294–304.

28. Cattoni F, Teté G, Calloni AM, et al. Milled versus moulded mock-ups based on the superimposition of 3D meshes from digital oral impressions: a comparative in vitro study in the aesthetic area. BMC Oral Health 2019;19(1):1–8.

29. Narang P, Shetty S, Prasad K. An in vivo study to determine the range of posterior teeth disclusion on working side in canine-guided occlusion. Indian J Dent Res 2012;23(6):814.

30. Kerstein RB. Reducing chronic masseter and temporalis muscular hyperactivity with computer-guided occlusal adjustments. Compend Contin Educ Dent 2010; 31(7):530–4.

31. Dawson PE. Envelope of function, Functional occlusion-e-book: from TMJ to smile design. Canada: Isevier Health Sciences; 2006. p. 141–8.

32. Lepidi L, Galli M, Mastrangelo F, et al. Virtual articulators and virtual mounting procedures: where do we stand? J Prosthodont 2021;30(1):24–35.

33. Londono J, Ghasemi S, Lawand G, et al. Evaluation of the golden proportion in the natural dentition: A systematic review and meta-analysis. J Prosthet Dent 2021;(S0022-3913-7). doi: S0022-3913(21)00415-7, In press.

34. Liao P, Fan Y, Nathanson D. Evaluation of maxillary anterior teeth width: a systematic review. J Prosthet Dent 2019;122(3):275–81, e7.

35. Akl MA, Mansour DE, Mays K, et al. Mathematical tooth proportions: a systematic review. J Prosthodont 2021. https://doi.org/10.1111/jopr.13420. In press.

36. Ward DH. Proportional smile design: using the recurring esthetic dental proportion to correlate the widths and lengths of the maxillary anterior teeth with the size of the face. Dental Clin 2015;59(3):623–38.

37. Nimbalkar S, Oh YY, Mok RY, et al. Smile attractiveness related to buccal corridor space in 3 different facial types: a perception of 3 ethnic groups of malaysians. J Prosthet Dent 2018;120(2):252–6.

38. Mollabashi V, Abolvardi M, Akhlaghian M, et al. Smile attractiveness perception regarding buccal corridor size among different facial types. Dental Med Probl 2018;55(3):305–12.

39. Oshagh M, Zarif NH, Bahramnia F. Evaluation of the effect of buccal corridor size on smile attractiveness. Eur J Esthet Dent 2010;5(4):370–80.

40. Cheng C-W, Ye S-Y, Chien C-H, et al. Randomized clinical trial of a conventional and a digital workflow for the fabrication of interim crowns: an evaluation of treatment efficiency, fit, and the effect of clinician experience. J Prosthet Dent 2021; 125(1):73–81.

41. Khanna N. The envelope of function: understanding and importance, . Functional Aesthetic Dentistry. 1st. Switzerland: Springer; 2020. p. 35–53. https://doi.org/10.1007/978-3-030-39115-7_3.

42. UTZ KH, Müller F, Lückerath W, et al. The lateral leeway in the habitual intercuspation: experimental studies and literature review. J Oral Rehabil 2007;34(6): 406–13.

43. Myagmar G, Lee J-H, Ahn J-S, et al. Wear of 3D printed and CAD/CAM milled interim resin materials after chewing simulation. J Adv Prosthodont 2021; 13(3):144.

44. Afrashtehfar KI, Bryant SR. Understanding the lived experience of north american dental patients with a single-tooth implant in the upper front region of the mouth: protocol for a qualitative study. JMIR Res Protoc 2021;10(6):e25767.

45. Gamer S, Tuch R, Garcia LT. MM House mental classification revisited: Intersection of particular patient types and particular dentist's needs. J Prosthet Dent 2003;89(3):297–302.

46. Mörch C, Atsu S, Cai W, et al. Artificial intelligence and ethics in dentistry: a scoping review. J Dent Res 2021;100(13):1452–60.

47. Revilla-León M, Gómez-Polo M, Vyas S, et al. Artificial intelligence models for tooth-supported fixed and removable prosthodontics: a systematic review. J Prosthet Dent 2021. doi: S0022-3913(21)00309-7, In press.

48. Revilla-León M, Gómez-Polo M, Vyas S, et al. Artificial intelligence applications in restorative dentistry: a systematic review. J Prosthet Dent 2021. doi: S0022-3913(21)00087-1, In press.

49. Chen Y-w, Stanley K, Att W. Artificial intelligence in dentistry: current applications and future perspectives. Quintessence Int 2020;51(3):248–57.

50. Touati R, Richert R, Millet C, et al. Comparison of two innovative strategies using augmented reality for communication in aesthetic dentistry: a pilot study. J Healthc Eng 2019;2019.

51. Fallahi HR, Keyhan SO, Cheshmi B, et al. Augmented reality: new horizons in oral and maxillofacial surgery, . Integrated procedures in facial cosmetic surgery. 1st. Switzerland: Springer; 2021. p. 593–7. https://doi.org/10.1007/978-3-030-46993-1_51.

52. Rodríguez CP, Judge RB, Castle D, et al. Body dysmorphia in dentistry and prosthodontics: a practice based study. J Dent 2019;81:33–8.

53. Panossian AJ, Block MS. Evaluation of the smile: facial and dental considerations. J Oral Maxillofac Surg 2010;68(3):547–54.

Smile Management
A Discussion with the Masters

Behnam Bohluli, DMD, FRCD(C)[a],*, Seied Omid Keyhan, DDS, OMFS[b,c],
André P. Saadoun, DMD, MS[d], Tatakis Dimitris, DDS, PhD[e],
Edward McLaren, DMD[f], Francesco Luigi Mintrone, DMD[g],
Neophytos Demetriades, DDS, MD, MSc[h], Seong-Gon Kim, DDS, PhD[i],
Shohreh Ghasemi, DMD[j], Martin Kasir, MD[k]

KEYWORDS

• Smile design • Gummy smile • Smile management

KEY POINTS

• The experts discuss some of the common challenging smile designs.
• The experts explain how they approach the complicated smile management cases.
• The experts explain how to avoid and manage complications.
• Finally, the experts discuss the recent advances and the future of smile design.

INTRODUCTION

Smile design is an ongoing challenge in both dentistry and facial cosmetics surgery. Herein, some very common smile design scenarios are shared with six world known masters. Each case will be reviewed by 2 cosmetic dentists, 2 periodontists, and 2

[a] Oral and Maxillofacial Surgery, University of Toronto, 124 Edward Street, Toronto ON, M5G 1G6, Canada; [b] College of Dentistry, Gangneung-Wonju National University, Gangneung, South Korea; [c] Department of Oral & Maxillofacial Surgery, University of Florida, College of Medicine, Jaksonville, FL, USA; [d] Diplomate, American Academy of Periodontology; Diplomate of the International Congress of Oral Implantologists; Private Practice limited to Esthetic Periodontics and Implant Surgery, Paris, France; [e] Division of Periodontology, College of Dentistry, The Ohio State University, Columbus, OH, USA; [f] Private practice, Park City, Utah; [g] Department of Dentistry and Oral Maxillo Facial Surgery, University of Modena and Reggio Emilia, Modena (MO), Italy; [h] Oral and Maxillofacial Surgery, European University of Cyprus School of Medicine, Facial Plastic and Reconstructive Surgery, European University of Cyprus School of Medicine, Nicosia, Cyprus; [i] Department of Oral and Maxillofacial Surgery, College of Dentistry, Gangneung-Wonju National University, Gangneung, 25457, Republic of Korea; [j] Department of Oral and Maxillofacial surgery, The Dental College of Georgia at Augusta University, Augusta, GA, USA; [k] Worldwide Laser Institute, Dallas, Texas, USA
* Corresponding author.
E-mail address: bbohluli@yahoo.com

Dent Clin N Am 66 (2022) 489–501
https://doi.org/10.1016/j.cden.2022.03.004
0011-8532/22/© 2022 Elsevier Inc. All rights reserved.

oral and maxillofacial surgeons. At the end, contributors will describe current advances and future prospects of this evolving field.

Behnam Bohluli: A 25-year-old healthy woman (**Fig. 1**) is willing to have smile improvements. She has seen many professionals and is very confused and disappointed. Her dentist believes she needs aesthetic crown lengthening and veneers for her front teeth. A dermatologist has advised *Botulinum* toxin injections, and her oral and maxillofacial surgeon has diagnosed her with *long face syndrome* and suggested jaw surgery. How can you help this group of patients find the best treatment plan?

André P. Saadoun: Advice Based on the Exposure of the Gingiva Less than 8 mm

- Establish the diagnosis: Is it a natural passive eruption type 1-A or a delayed passive eruption type 1-B?
- Orthodontic treatment to realign the teeth, increase the width of the arches, and ingress the teeth by 1 to 2 mm.
- Digital face/smile analysis, workflow surgical guide to perform precisely the crown lengthening.
- Placement of a PMA block in the maxillary upper concavity before closing the full-thickness flap to limit the upper lip muscles contractions.
- Oral hygiene maintenance personal and professional.

Tatakis Dimitris

My advice to patients who find themselves in a similar situation would be to ask their health care provider or providers all the right questions, which should include questions regarding the reasons for the choice of the proposed treatment, the expected short- and long-term outcomes, possible complications, and potential alternatives. Furthermore, the patients need to ask to see examples of cases treated in the proposed manner, to be able to ascertain whether a similar outcome would be satisfactory to them. I would also encourage the patients to express in detail which specific aspect, or aspects, of their smile is of most concern to them.

Edward McLaren

With this limited source of information, our first evaluation would be to assess how much the upper lip moves when the patient makes a normal smile. My guess is her upper lip is moving about 12 to 14 mm, and clearly, she has a global diagnosis of a gummy smile.

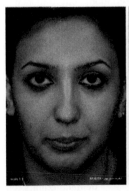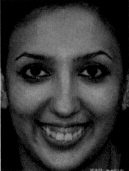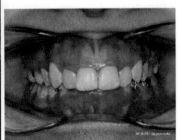

Fig. 1. Long face syndrome.

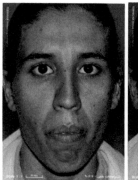
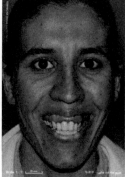
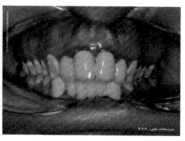

Fig. 2. Complications after aesthetic crown lengthening and crowns for the front teeth.

There are several basic causes of a gummy smile.

- One cause is the hypermobile upper lip. Typically, we would like to see 8 to 9 mm of upper lip movement in a normal smile. My guess is that her upper lip moves somewhere around 12 or 13 mm from the lip at rest to full smile.
- The other cause of a gummy smile is vertical maxillary excess. It means that the whole maxilla is incisally displaced. In these patients, it looks like someone with a denture that is falling down in the mouth.

Here, it clearly looks like vertical maxillary excess is a component of her face. Up until now, at least 2 things are going on here, and 2 of the 4 possible diagnoses of a gummy smile are evident.

We also look at the 2 actual sizes of the tooth and reference where the cementoenamel junction (CEJ) is. We want to know where that is relative to the gingival margin because it could be a component we called delayed passive eruption. We want to know where that free gingival margin is again relative to the CEJ, so I'm guessing she has a little bit of that too. We probably could easily move the soft tissue of about 2 mm and get it to the CEJ. One of the recommendations is crown lengthening. I do not like to do crown lengthening for aesthetic reasons beyond the CEJ. I do not want to

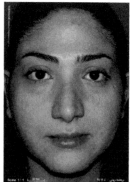
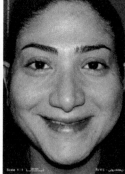
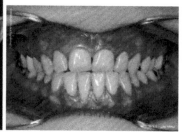

Fig. 3. Lacking smile components.

expose a root surface because it causes potential problems down the road. Therefore, I am guessing we could get 1.5 or 2 mm of the gum safely biologically.

In brief, her maxilla is significantly incisally displaced, and my treatment plan would be a strong discussion with the orthodontist and maxillofacial surgery team to impact the maxilla. I think one of my primary recommendations is to have orthognathic surgery performed.

I usually consider the least-invasive treatment plans, and I guess you could not call maxillofacial surgery a noninvasive procedure. Meanwhile, these surgeries are done so well today by surgeons that the results are predictable and the morbidity from it is practically zero. I would do all that first and then reevaluate maybe with a little bleaching and a little bit of aesthetic recontouring of the teeth possibly, and see if that does not satisfy her needs. Then, we can always do the veneers at the end.

Now, what if she refuses, and if she says NO? No way I am going to do all of those procedures. Let us talk about just doing the crown lengthening up to the CEJ and not expose the roots. I could do that in Photoshop for her, and I could show her what she would looks like in Photoshop and then reshape the teeth a little bit to get a better balance; or, you know, what if we go up 2 mm here and get to the CEJ, then you know she is only showing maybe 3 to 3.5 mm of soft tissue. Then, from there, there are some other procedures that may help as an adjunct. Because she does have a hypermobile upper lip, we can put a little botulinum toxin in there to see if that works.

The other effective procedure may be lip repositioning. A pie-shaped piece of soft tissue is removed, and the lip is tied and repositioned so that the upper lip cannot move as much.

Francesco Luigi Mintrone

Here, with current information, it is very difficult to make a proper diagnosis because we need cephalometric data to analyze the jaws and the teeth.

In my opinion, the mandible is not in the ideal position; the patient is class II and has a clear deep bite. Therefore, it seems that the first treatment is orthodontic treatment. It is obvious that in these situations a gummy smile cannot be corrected by crown lengthening. I believe veneers are not also indicated for her. In brief, I believe she is not a prosthodontics case, and I would suggest orthodontic treatment and probably orthognathic surgery, and finally, bleaching, and nothing else.

Neophytos Demetriades

For every patient who presents to our office for cosmetic evaluation, we should initially ask them to explain and determine their main cosmetic concern. However, the cosmetic surgeon is a responsible expert in evaluating the face, recognizing and diagnosing the underlying disease and the cause of the cosmetic problem, and providing to the patient the appropriate treatment. For the patient in **Fig. 1**, who suffers from a cosmetic gummy smile, the borderline disease is a maxillofacial, skeletal malocclusion with vertical maxillary excess, and the appropriate treatment to correct the smile should be a combination of an orthodontic and orthognathic surgery treatment. Of course, botulinum toxin can give a temporary solution, but it will not correct all the aspects of this defective smile. All the above should be explained to the patient, and all the options should be given before any treatment.

Seong-Gon Kim

This patient showed (1) upper lip length to lower lip length ratio was almost 1 and (2) a deep bite. As her upper lip length was relatively long for lower lip length, there would be little benefit from botulinum toxin injection. Maxillary alveolar bone excess was also evident. The occlusal plane seemed to be steep. Thus, the primary treatment option would be the anterior segmental osteotomy. If the patient does not like surgical treatment, then the second option would be orthodontic intrusion of maxillary anterior teeth using the skeletal anchorage system. In the case of the second option, periodontal surgery, such as crown lengthening, should be considered as a supplementary treatment.

Shohreh Ghasemi

My advice is based on the display of the gingiva less than 8 mm and measuring the width and thickness of attached gingiva, CEJ, and probing depth.

- The treatment modalities vary according to the cause of the gummy smile.
- The key is accurately recognizing the cause of the pathologic condition. In some cases, the gummy smile results from more than one factor, for example, vertical maxillary excess and hypermobile lip, and a combination of techniques can be implemented. Less-invasive treatment options include botulin toxin injection and a newer alternative technique with hyaluronic acid infiltration into the paranasal region. It requires a vast knowledge of anatomy owing to the vascular region. Another option is LipStaT, which is a versatile technique to achieve the ideal result. Oral hygiene can be reinstated after 48 hours, and the results are noticeable as early as 1 week after the procedure and maintained at follow-up visits.

Martin Kasir

I think she clearly has hyperfunctioning lip elevators, and botulinum toxin would be an easy start for her, easy and with no downtime. Her status could then be reevaluated.

Omid Keyhan: a young woman (**Fig. 2**) has undergone aesthetic crown lengthening and crowns for the front teeth. What is your general recommendation to avoid these complications?

André P. Saadoun: Advice Based on the Exposure of the Gingiva More than 8 mm

- Establish the diagnosis: Is it a natural passive eruption type 1-A or a delayed passive eruption type 1-B?
- Maxillary orthognathic surgery, type Le Fort 1 staying 2 mm from the apex of the anterior teeth and ALSO decreasing the chin height (that will decrease the long face syndrome)
- Scaling, root planning, and patient hygiene reinforcement
- Remove old crown Rastafarians, place new temporary crowns
- A few months after the orthogenetic surgery on the maxillary, workflow surgical guide to harmonize the gingival contours and reestablish a perfect biological width of 2.5 to 3 mm from the new teeth preparation
- Three to 6 months after soft tissue healing, build up new restorations in harmony with the esthetic gingival level and the new smile

Tatakis Dimitris

To avoid these complications, it is necessary to approach each case with a proper and complete diagnostic protocol. This will help accurately establish the cause or causes underlying the presenting condition and appropriately guide the treatment. In addition, the indicated/chosen treatment must be executed correctly and to a high standard.

Edward McLaren

The first thing that you want to do in this person is remove the from the teeth and get some decent provisionals for prototypes to get this tissue healthy.

Then, the next thing is going to be a similar sort of treatment as recommended by the first case. It is a maxillofacial orthodontics case. That method is the main way we are going to treat this case: get everything aligned, widen the arch form a little bit, and then level the gingiva as best as possible.

This patient also has long face syndrome. Therefore, orthognathic surgery to impact the maxilla may be followed, and then possibly, a couple of implants can be placed in the lower jaw to solve some problems. Then, it is hard to tell without looking in person, but the patient may have some structural and biologic problems with the teeth up top that might need to be addressed. The patient may possibly need extractions and implants, so she will be a very difficult case that will require multidisciplinary efforts. I am sure every form of discipline is going to be needed on this case to solve this problem.

Francesco Luigi Mintrone

In similar cases, I would start with cephalometric analysis to make the proper treatment plan. Meanwhile, it is evident that this patient is an orthographic surgery case and has not had an appropriate indication for a crown-lengthening procedure. Currently, the crowns are not precise and have caused inflammation. The crown lengthening has not been done properly, and only the anterior teeth are involved in the crown-lengthening procedure to correct the gummy smile. It is clear that in addition to orthodontic treatment and orthographic surgery, the problems caused by previous treatment should be corrected as much as possible, and periodontal surgery and prosthodontics treatments would be recommended.

Neophytos Demetriades

In order to avoid these complications, every patient should be evaluated thoroughly, and a premade protocol of evaluation should be followed by the cosmetic surgeon. Sometimes, if we have a constructive, organized, and protocolized evaluation, we can understand and diagnose the underlying diseases that may cause the cosmetic defect. A collaboration with specialists from other specialties may be necessary before we finalize our treatment and proceed with any kind of surgery. For this patient, it is obvious by the pictures that she suffers from skeletal malocclusion, and furthermore, if we evaluate the lips on a closed mouth position, there is lip stretching indicating vertical maxillary excess. In addition, the length of the upper lip seems to be adequate (no lip incompetency), and the length of the crowns of the anterior teeth seems to be long enough with no indication of short crowns or overgrowth gingiva. This is a patient that will benefit maximally from orthognathic surgery.

Seong-Gon Kim

When the patient was in the resting position, the hyperactive chin muscle was found. As I do not have the lateral cephalometric view, she might have bimaxillary protrusion. Although prosthodontic treatment with periodontal surgery has shown a certain effect on limited cases of the gummy smile, it will have a very limited therapeutic effect on the bimaxillary protrusion. The primary treatment option for this patient may be Le Fort I osteotomy with mandibular surgery. In the case of the Le Fort I osteotomy, superior impaction with correcting the occlusal plane angle will be required.

Shohreh Ghasemi

The main and crucial issue for consideration of gingivectomy is the amount of biological width. A gingivectomy can be successful when there are adequate osseous levels and attached gingiva, and the gingival tissue from bone to gingival crest is more than 3 mm. However, a full-thickness periodontal flap in combination with osteotomy is indicated when the osseous level is near the cementoenamel junction, and a gingivectomy alone will disrupt the biologic width. It is essential to differentiate between the conditions that cause the gingival overexposure.

Four to 6 months after surgical treatment, referral to the restorative dentist can be beneficial to harmonize the dental proportion for achievement of the best smile design.

Behnam Bohluli: A 27-year-old woman (**Fig. 3**) needs smile improvement. In contrast to most smile design cases, she lacks smile components. What are your treatment options for this type of problem?

André P. Saadoun

My advice is based on the exposure of the gingiva, and in this case, one almost does not see the patient's teeth, because it is an upper low lip line showing as much as 25% to 50% of the maxillary anterior patient's smile! Furthermore, her lower lip and chin have strong muscles, which increase the crown teeth disappearance.

The diagnosis, which shows that it is a very difficult and not a usual case compared with the excess of gingival exposure, is always treated in general with a crown-lengthening procedure and with other therapy.

It would be interesting to check if there is a tongue interposition during the deglutition.

Because of her short upper lip when she smiles, it not possible to recommend the new technique of raising apically the upper lip surgically.

As a periodontist clinician, I would refer her to an oral surgeon to take care of the chin in order to decrease the height, modify the shape from a triangle to a round shape, and release some pertinent muscles.

Then, the patient should be referred to an orthodontist to increase the vertical dimension by 2 to 3 mm by egressing all the maxillary teeth.

At the end of that orthodontic phase, there will be a reevaluation of the smile, and maybe a limited crown lengthening should be recommended if it is a delayed passive eruption with uneven gingival contour; some laminate veneers could achieve the esthetic of this new smile to show more of her smile.

Tatakis Dimitris

The clinical images suggest normal soft tissues (upper lip) and dentoalveolar anomalies, including malocclusion, in the anterior dentition. Orthodontic consultation would be the first option in this type of problem, followed by oral and maxillofacial surgery evaluation for possible orthognathic treatment needs and periodontal assessment to address the potential future need for aesthetic crown lengthening after completion of orthodontic treatment.

Edward McLaren

I would obviously have a periodontal consultation to see if any procedure is needed before orthodontic treatment and then would continue with orthodontic treatment. She has a bit of a strong chin, so orthognathic surgery needs to be considered.

In brief, I recommend definitely a periodontal consultation and then orthodontic consultation. This will probably be finished up with veneers just because I do not like aesthetical proportions and the shape of the teeth.

Francesco Luigi Mintrone

This patient needs a multidisciplinary approach. Here, the upper jaw seems to be atrophic, and it seems that maxilla needs to be longer and more forward in position. The plan is to start with orthodontic treatment. Then, the analysis will show if orthographic surgery would be needed. In my opinion, the teeth look fine, and there is no need for aggressive prosthodontics intervention. After orthodontic treatment and orthognathic surgery, minimally invasive prosthodontic procedures, such as veneers, may be advocated.

Neophytos Demetriades

The clinical images suggest a patient with normal length of the upper lip, no teeth show at smile, deep buccal corridor, and mild protrusion of the chin. In addition, it seems that the patient has undergone rhinoplasty; however, there is no support of the columella with collapsed columella owing to the lack of support from the anterior nasal spine. In my opinion, this is a class III patient, as can be seen by the intraoral picture, with maxillary hypoplasia. In addition, she may have a short crown of the anterior teeth. I believe this patient will be benefit from orthodontic treatment initially, followed by orthognathic surgery, which will advance the maxilla forward and correct the occlusal plane to give more maxillary teeth show and correct at the same time the overbite.

Seong-Gon Kim

The patient shows the edge bite with a class III malocclusion. She has a reverse smile line and insufficient maxillary vertical dimension. A mild level of lower gingival recession was also found. When she smiled, a hyperactive chin muscle was found. To correct her smile line, orthognathic surgery with orthodontic treatment would be required. Decompensation of occlusion would be required before orthognathic surgery. In the case of orthognathic surgery, Le Fort I osteotomy for posterior impaction and ramus osteotomy for mandibular setback would be required. If she does not like surgery, she may be treated by extraction of the 4 premolars and orthodontic treatment.

Shohreh Ghasemi

My advice is based on the lack of gingival display in the smile. It is a restorative challenge to achieve ideal esthetics. My advice is to use a gingivectomy or laser-assisted gingival contouring procedure. However, this simplistic approach can potentially create a mucogingival defect or a biological width violation. To avoid these periodontal-restorative complications, it is important during treatment planning to assess the anatomic relationship that resulted in the gummy smile and choose the appropriate surgical treatment to eliminate this condition.

OMID KEYHAN: WHAT HAS CHANGED IN YOUR SMILE MANAGEMENT DURING THE PAST 5 YEARS?

André P. Saadoun

As in any cosmetic intervention, the therapeutic objectives must be clearly defined beforehand, between the clinician and the patient and in correlation with the analysis of the initial clinical situation. This will allow the clinician to give a scientific classification and then a clinical diagnosis, and therefore, the most and best adapted treatment for this specific patient.

The patient should be perfectly informed about the preoperative, perioperative, and postoperative steps and sign a consent form before starting any treatment!

The utilization of the cone-beam computed tomography (CBCT), the Computer-Aided Design/Computer-Aided Manufacturing (CAD/CAM), the digital face/smile design, the analysis, and the digital workflow have change dramatically the crown-lengthening procedures, by using a surgical guide defining the amount and marginal gingiva and bone crest by ostectomy, and osteoplasty to remove.

Another surgical change modality has been the surgical coronal repositioning of the upper lip by making a line of incision at 1 mm below the MG junction and then by removing a certain but precise quantity of alveolar mucosa inside the upper vestibule, before suturing the new upper line of incision to the border of the keratinized gingiva close to the MGJ, that will decrease the amount of the upper lip mobility and teeth exposure.

Lately, the utilization of fillers and botulinum toxin could limit the upper lips' hyper-mobility and movement during normal and forced smile mobility, which bring us to the next question.

Tatakis Dimitris

There has been a gradual shift to consistently consider less-invasive surgical options, such as lip repositioning, in cases of excessive gingival display owing to a hypermobile upper lip.

Edward McLaren

Nothing. I am sure other people think that I am the first one to come up with using Photoshop back in 2002 for doing smile designs. I still use Photoshop. Obviously, Photoshop evolved to the multiple-level new versions that make the process of smile design so much easier.

The other principle that I use in smile design concepts is something that I learned a long time ago, maybe 20 years ago or even longer, which is conservative treatment, and I am still being very conservative.

SO, NOTHING HAS CHANGED FOR ME IN THE PAST FIVE YEARS.

Francesco Luigi Mintrone

In my own practice, I am turning more and more to the digital world. In the past few years, I have had the opportunity to prepare a 3-dimensional (3D) design of the smile of the patient with a great precision, and with this approach, I can show the final results to the patient before starting the treatment. This gives the chance to assess the treatment plan with the patient and discuss the possible alternatives.

Neophytos Demetriades

Over the years, I developed a protocol that is followed as a basic evaluation for every patient who comes to me with smile concerns. Following this protocol, I realized that many patients with different smile defects suffer from an underlying skeletal malocclusion. In addition, older patients go through a progressive age-related lengthening of the upper lip. In this group of patients, a lip lift approach is indicated to correct their smile problem more than any injection of fillers, which may worsen the existing smile defect.

Seong-Gon Kim

For the maxillofacial surgeon, an unattractive smile of surgical patients is a consequence of skeletal discrepancy. Many patients having skeletal malocclusion showed an unattractive smile. These patients have been considered an orthognathic candidate. Recently, there have been many advancements in the skeletal anchorage system and in the application of botulinum toxin. Dental intrusion using the skeletal anchorage system has been used for improving the gummy smile. The amount of intrusion obtained by the skeletal anchorage system has been reported from 1.92 mm to 6 mm. However, high incidence of root resorption is a complication of dental intrusion using the skeletal anchorage system. The application of botulinum toxin is a relatively safe and simple procedure. However, the effect of injection is transient, and the indication is limited. Furthermore, the purpose of botulinum toxin injection is an inducing nonfunctional state of upper lip elevating muscles like myotomy. Despite limited success in covering upper gingiva, the smile itself is unnatural.

For the successful smile management, the precise diagnosis is a vital component. The problem list should be individualized by the parameters that can define natural smile. There have been some changes in correcting the unattractive smile without skeletal discrepancy, and most changes have happened in orthodontics, periodontics, and prosthodontics. However, orthognathic surgery has been still the primary option for correcting the unattractive smile with skeletal discrepancy.

Shohreh Ghasemi

A fundamental objective of an aesthetic treatment is the patient's satisfaction in the last 10 years, and that the outcome of the treatment should meet the patient's expectation of enhancing his/her facial aesthetics and smile. A patient constantly doubting the result of the treatment, which is an irreversible procedure, can be motivated and educated through Digital Smile Designing (DSD) technique. DSD is a technical tool that is used to design and modify the smile of patients digitally and help them to visualize it beforehand by creating and presenting a digital mockup of their new smile design before the treatment physically starts. It helps in visual communication and involvement of the patients in their own smile design process, thus ensuring predictable treatment outcome and increasing case acceptance.

Designing an aesthetic smile is a complex process that can be approached by collaboration with different specialties, and combination therapies with the aspects of digital smile and facial aesthetic treatment with filler and botulinum toxin for improvement of excessive upper lip mobility, and aesthetic dentistry will enhance the advantages and prospects.

Martin Kasir

I have actually become more conservative with smile management. I refer more patients to my periodontist colleagues for corrective gum surgery as outlined above. Also, I have become MORE conservative with upper lip fillers, as I feel overfilling the upper lip can have a negative effect on the patient's smile. Finally, the new procedure called Lip Lifting has taken off, which helps correct longer upper lips and to evert flattened upper lips.

BEHNAM BOHLULI: WHAT DO YOU THINK ABOUT THE FUTURE OF SMILE DESIGN?
André P. Saadoun

There are many crown-lengthening surgical techniques, and they are dependent on the initial situation and the objectives to achieve.

Establishing an adequate classification, and a correct diagnosis, based on the Coslet and colleagues[1] publication regarding the amount of keratinized gingiva (type I for a large quantity of keratinized gingiva and type II for a short quantity of keratinized gingiva) and the CEJ location in relation to the cervical bone crest (subtype A with 1.5 mm distance or more and subtype B at 0 mm to 0.5 mm) would definitely help the clinician to choose the most appropriate surgical procedure to restore the normal biological width at the end of each surgical session between the natural passive eruption and the altered passive eruption.

This surgical concept will prevent the recurrence of soft tissue rebound over the teeth, esthetic complications, and certainly achieve an optimal long-term esthetic result.

The utilization of CBCT, the CAD CAM, the digital face/smile design analysis, and the digital workflow have changed dramatically the crown-lengthening procedures, especially for the gingival smile management, establishing a more precise smile design and a diagnosis and using also a digital surgical guide to perform the surgery in a more precise and minimally invasive approach and give self-confidence to the patient who could prefigure in advance the final esthetic periodontal and functional result.

Today, the amount of gingiva exposure on smiling and forced smile will determine more predictably what will be the best options for the patient and the clinical specialist to be consulted.

One should consider the following:

- An exposure of 2 to 4 mm could be handled first by a periodontist with maybe the input of an orthodontist.
- An exposure between 4 and 8 mm could be handled by an orthodontist and a cosmetic surgeon with fillers and botulinum toxin, and the final touch handled by a periodontist.
- An exposure of more than 8 mm would be handled by an orthognathic surgeon, with the help of a combination of an orthodontic, a cosmetic specialist, and a periodontist to harmonize the gingival level with respect to the teeth proportion.
- Some restorative work, such as laminated veneers or crowns, may be necessary to finalize this long and complex treatment plan.

Tatakis Dimitris

Like many other aspects of what we do clinically, the future of smile design will incorporate more digital approaches and solutions, especially from a diagnostic and treatment planning perspective.

Edward McLaren

I think in the future we are going to have very interactive live 3D smile designs where we can scan the patients while they are moving around, and then we can actually create a 3D rendering of where we want the bone, the soft tissue, and the teeth. This will help show the patient in real time what they will look like. It will be similar to the things we see with the programs to buy sunglasses. Thereafter, I think that will be a big benefit, and then from there, the algorithm programs can be written to show us where the teeth are now, where the gingiva is now, and where you would like it to be. In addition, we will easily find out what is involved to achieve these goals. The point is that we will know those things before we get too deep into the treatment plan.

Francesco Luigi Mintrone

Right now, we are using advanced technologies in our practice. Therefore, the base will remain almost the same. Meanwhile, in the future, a team approach, including a cosmetic dentist, an orthodontist, and a laboratory technician will be the mainstay of smile management.

Neophytos Demetriades

I believe in the future a more solidified protocol of smile evaluation will appear, and a standardized clinical evaluation of smile will be developed, which will indicate the appropriate treatment, which will involve many specialists from different specialties. More understanding of the skeletal malocclusion and the effect that has on a proper smile along with the lengthening of the upper lip through age will dictate more specific surgical procedures that will provide better results to the patients with smile defects.

Seong-Gon Kim

The definition of an attractive smile is influenced by historical, cultural, and demographic background. The prevalent smile style is also different to study groups. Upward lip curvature is prevalent in Pakistan. However, straight lip curvature is prevalent in China. Therefore, the ideal treatment plan for the attractive smile should be tailored to the individual preference. The individual preference will determine the future of smile design.

There has still been limitation in correcting the unattractive smile without orthognathic surgery. As smile design is a highly delicate process, a precise treatment plan and surgery are important for the successful treatment. Three-dimensional modeling using computer-aided design and manufacturing has been widely used in the orthognathic surgery. Surgical template and prebended plate can help to make precise bone-cut with positioning. The ultrasonic bone scalpel can cut the interdental bone without root and soft tissue damage. These emerging technologies will make it possible to achieve a reliable surgical outcome.

Shohreh Ghasemi

Over the last few decades, cosmetic dentistry has become increasingly commonplace as more and more Americans look for a healthier, prettier smile. In recent years, advanced technologies and decreasing cost have helped make treatment affordable for a diverse range of budgets.

Cosmetic dentistry is increasingly becoming an issue of concern to patients who hope to improve their smile. A systematic and comprehensive dentofacial analysis must be performed before commencing esthetic treatment. Golden proportion, soft tissue measurement, smile and smile line assessment, orofacial indexes and scales, incisor proportion and angulation, and facial esthetics. These categories included various esthetic parameters, including the smile line, lip line, incisal offset, location of dental and facial midline, incisor angulations and width to height ratios of the maxillary anterior teeth, gingival contour, and root coverage and papilla height. These parameters should be considered when providing dental treatment in the anterior area, as they allow for quantification and objective judgment.

Smile aesthetics is based on numerical, physical, physiologic, and psychological data regarding beauty, while considering the desires of the patient. It is determined by the shape, color, and position of the lips, teeth, and gingival tissues. Periodontal examination in both the facial and the labial settings supports analysis of the gingival display during natural and forced smiling, the health of the periodontium, the gingival contours, the aesthetic gingival line, and the presence of the papillae.

During implementation of the global orthodontic treatment plan, periodontal plastic surgery can change the gingival appearance and morphology in order to restore the harmony of the smile. Subtractive periodontal plastic surgery treats biological space defects and excess tissue during incomplete passive eruption by gingivectomy or apically positioned flap, combined, or not, with osteoplasty or osteotomy. Finally, injections of hyaluronic acid in the papillae can plump them up and minimize the size of any black holes.

Martin Kasir

I believe the future of smile design is clearly headed for collaboration between dentists and dermatologists. Most smiles can likely benefit from the help from both specialties, as a smile is not limited to only teeth, gums, vermilion, or cutaneous lip. The shape and size of the teeth and gums, together with the color, quality, and positioning of the cutaneous lip, all play a major role in a patient's smile.

REFERENCES

1. Coslet JG, Ingber JS, Rose LF, et al.The "biologic width"–a concept in periodontics and restorative dentistry. Alpha Omegan 1977;70(3):62–5.

FURTHER READINGS

Bastidas JA. Surgical Correction of the "Gummy Smile". Oral Maxillofacial Surg Clin N Am 2021;33:197–209.

McLaren EA, Rifkin R. Macroesthetics: facial and dentofacial analysis. J Calif Dent Assoc 2002;30(11):839–46.

McLaren EA, Goldstein RE. The Photoshop Smile Design Technique. Compend Contin Educ Dent 2018;39(5):e17–20.

Narita M, Takaki T, Shibahara T, et al. Utilization of desktop 3D printer-fabricated "Cost-Effective" 3D models in orthognathic surgery. Maxillofac Plast Reconstr Surg 2020;42:24.

Park SY, Hwang DS, Song JM, et al. Comparison of time and cost between conventional surgical planning and virtual surgical planning in orthognathic surgery in Korea. Maxillofac Plast Reconstr Surg 2021;43:18.

Silva CO, Rezende RI, Mazuquini AC, et al. Aesthetic crown lengthening and lip repositioning surgery: pre- and post-operative assessment of smile attractiveness. J Clin Periodontol 2021;48(6):826–33.

Silva CO, Ribeiro-Júnior NV, Campos TV, et al. Excessive gingival display: treatment by a modified lip repositioning technique. J Clin Periodontol 2013;40(3):260–5.

Silva CO, Soumaille JM, Marson FC, et al. Aesthetic crown lengthening: periodontal and patient-centred outcomes. J Clin Periodontol 2015;42(12):1126–s1134.

Moving?

Make sure your subscription moves with you!

To notify us of your new address, find your **Clinics Account Number** (located on your mailing label above your name), and contact customer service at:

Email: journalscustomerservice-usa@elsevier.com

800-654-2452 (subscribers in the U.S. & Canada)
314-447-8871 (subscribers outside of the U.S. & Canada)

Fax number: 314-447-8029

Elsevier Health Sciences Division
Subscription Customer Service
3251 Riverport Lane
Maryland Heights, MO 63043

*To ensure uninterrupted delivery of your subscription, please notify us at least 4 weeks in advance of move.

ELSEVIER

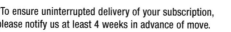